C000294854

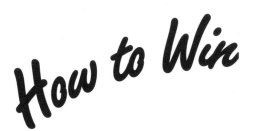

How to Win at Yoga

Nail the hardest poses and find your selfie

FEATURING:

@daretomove @litasattva @emilymergyoga @alanellmanyoga
@katarinarayburnyoga @natashacornishyoga @helenrussellclark
@nickiratcliffe @davjonesyoga @hannahwhittinghamyoga
@yogetoverit @cteagz @jonelleyoga @sylviasyoga
@kimbalbumstead @tomberryart @plastic_horse @catfordshuffle
@goodlordveda @anadiasyoga @naijaboybending @rachaldo
@notordinaryjoe @juan.montoliu @leonrocketlondon
@tomholmesembodied @isabelankesteryoga @model.family
@szwerink @ambrasana

Marcus Veda & Hannah Whittingham

Vermilion
LONDON

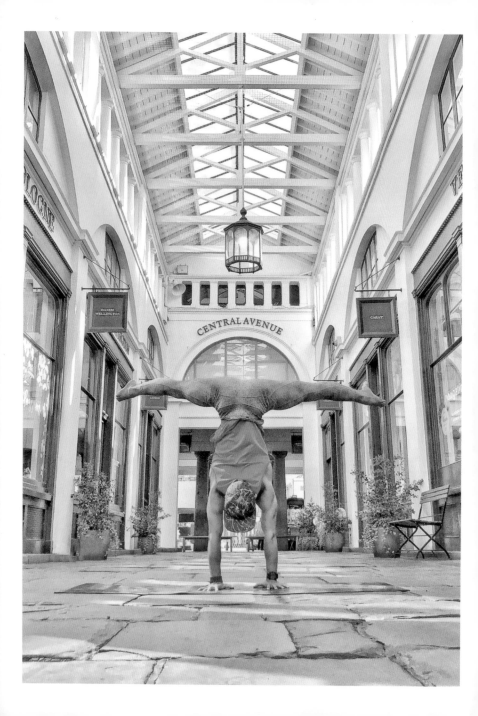

Contents

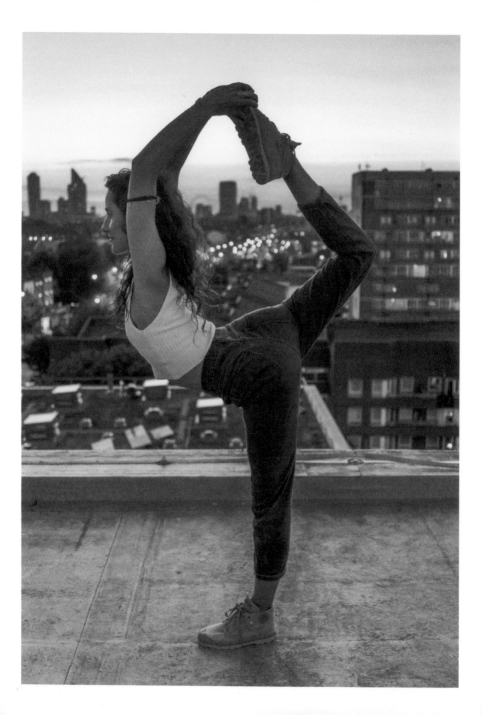

Introduction

Five years ago a few downward-facing Dogs, a standing tree and a seated meditation would have satisfied your average postural yoga class. Today it is becoming increasingly clear, both in class and online, that a lot of people wish to gain enlightenment through sticking their foot behind their head. Preferably in a handstand, ideally in the splits – and then take a picture.

Whether enlightenment is achievable through a one-legged flying pigeon or not (and whether enlightenment even matters if you didn't take a picture), crowded yoga studios are not the ideal place to test out your funky moves without the risk of your foot landing behind somebody else's head.

Lucky for you, this book is here to demystify some big poses: the ways in, the ways out, tips, drills, costume suggestions and ideal photogenic backdrops. So you can learn to win at yoga publicly, from the safety of your own space.*

* Technically, 'winning' is not something you can do at yoga, but on Instagram all yoga rules are void.

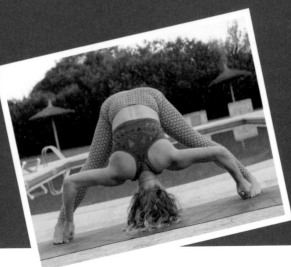

WHAT YOU WILL NEED

Other than a certain level of strength, a compliant skeleton, and patience of mind, you don't really need anything at all. The joy of yoga is that no fancy equipment is required, no expensive tools and no special clothes.*
A yoga mat can be useful though is not essential, and any equipment we think could help get you in and out of poses is laid out at the start of each section, followed by a list of household item substitutions, so you can assemble your armoury before you begin.

HOW TO USE THIS BOOK

Each pose begins with an indication of what's required of you: elements of flexibility, strength and stability that are essential to perform the pose safely.

If you already know that your hamstrings are so noodle-like you can fold yourself through your own legs, or your shoulders are so tight you haven't lifted your arms above your chest since 2005, then you can target which elements need more work right from the start. If you don't know, don't panic. Most people don't. Instead, work your way through the gateway poses, paying attention to which ones come easy and which ones prove something of a challenge. Your level of flexibility and strength will soon become apparent through your levels of sweat and your desire to swear loudly as you execute each one.

The gateway poses in each chapter are all designed to help you learn what needs a little work, as well as working towards the shape of the ultimate pose. Work through them in order, as often they will build on the one before.

* Does not apply to Instagram yoga.

Practise all of them regularly, but if one is especially difficult for you (and/or focusses on an area you know you need particular help with), then you can of course devote more of your time to it.

Your starting level of strength and flexibility will determine how long you'll need to practise before you tackle the final pose, but as a general rule, try to get to the stage where you can comfortably hold each gateway pose for the required time before you move on.

If you're ever confused by any of our terminology, there's a glossary of weird yoga terms and metaphors on p. 190 (so you can start bandying them about and confusing others with them too).

TIMESCALE

Many of these poses will take years of falling on your face, your nose and your houseplants before you master them, and what's more, how accessible each pose is to you will come down to your frame, your natural range of motion, and your current level of flexibility and strength. So be patient.

Practise as regularly as your schedule allows, keeping in mind that how frequently you work through the gateway poses and strengthening exercises will go a long way towards determining how soon the pose arrives, but also remembering that things like jobs, children, friendships and Netflix marathons are sometimes almost as important as handstands.

Try to accept defeat gracefully. If, after many months or years of working on your flexibility, you're still finding a particular full pose impossible to access, it may simply be that your bones aren't going to let you in.

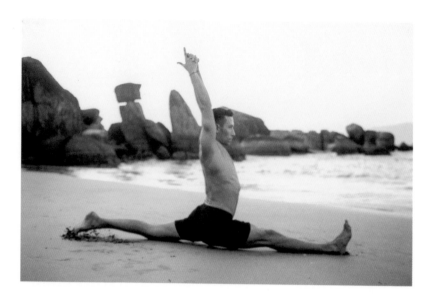

SAFETY

Yoga is not supposed to injure you. Listen to your body. Be kind and non-violent to yourself and to others, and never do anything that could hurt you, your housemates or your pets.

Although some of the stretching postures in this book will feel intense, the pain should never be sharp, so learn how to distinguish between stretchy pain and gone-too-far pain in your body. Be particularly careful around knees, hips, shoulders and the lower back, since these are areas often tweaked or pulled through over-zealous practice. Read our instructions carefully, and if you develop pain, or are working with an ongoing injury, always check in with a qualified body worker or physiotherapist to make sure you are OK to continue with these practices.

Kindness extends to your mental chatter, so talk nicely to yourself. Remember that every body is different, so your body may well look different in a posture to the pictures in this book. That is fine, and normal. You are special, so pay attention to how things feel rather than necessarily how they look.

Instagram yoga

Doing a handstand will not make you a better person – but doing a handstand, taking a picture, then putting it on Instagram at the perfect time of day with all the appropriate hashtags will make you an enormously popular person. Which is of course what life is all about.

For the Instayogis who know that perfectly proportioned pictures are where #samadhi (bliss) lies, after each technical run-down we will make suggestions on those vital aspects of yoga like costume, location, props, and how to pass your selfie off as an inspirational piece of life advice.

HASHTAGS & INSPOSLOGANS

Perhaps the most important element of your Insta post is successfully passing off a selfie as a piece of life-changing advice. You can do this by adding an inspirational quote either on the picture or in the text beneath.

Quotes from Rumi work particularly well. As do words from the Buddha, multiple examples of which can be found with a quick internet search. (NB It is not necessary to understand the original context of a quote to use it as a caption for your pose.)

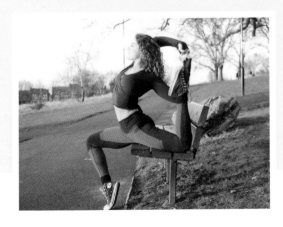

INSTA-READY

As well as all your physical preparation for each of the poses, you'll need to make sure of the following:

You have worked out how to use the timer on your iPhone and/or bribed a friend or partner to be your photographer. If the latter, in keeping with the Instagram by-laws, make sure you credit them with a camera emoji at the end of each post. (This way they have little choice but to 'Like' it.)

Make sure you have sufficient memory space on your phone. Do not expect the first 10 or 80 photos to be The One. You will likely need to take a large number before retiring to a gloomy room out of the sun to examine them forensically before you post.

Finally, visit your locations before you shoot them in order to work out where the sun will rise and set, and always have someone on hand for crowd control, mainly to shout the photo-bombers (tourists/animals/clouds) out of your shot before you snap.

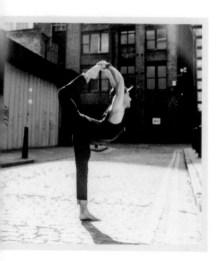

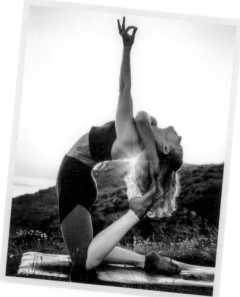

Body Guide

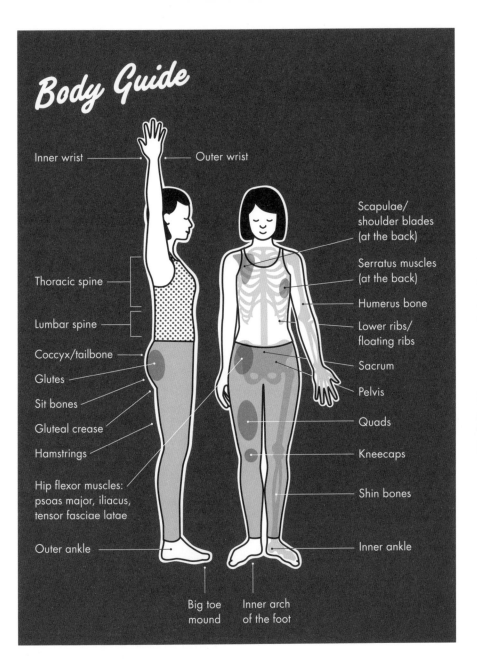

Inner wrist — Outer wrist

Thoracic spine

Lumbar spine

Coccyx/tailbone

Glutes

Sit bones

Gluteal crease

Hamstrings

Hip flexor muscles: psoas major, iliacus, tensor fasciae latae

Outer ankle

Scapulae/ shoulder blades (at the back)

Serratus muscles (at the back)

Humerus bone

Lower ribs/ floating ribs

Sacrum

Pelvis

Quads

Kneecaps

Shin bones

Inner ankle

Big toe mound

Inner arch of the foot

HANUMANASANA

1

Full Splits

Hanumanasana, or the front splits, can be practised in many incarnations, from split backbends and leg catches to standing splits with your leg up by your ear. In this instance we will be looking at the square-hipped, on-the-ground, active-legged Hanumanasana, for the simple reason that it's a useful pose.

Although the need to split your legs to 180 degrees is rarely called for in 'civilian' life, a well-executed splits can do many things to help your body go about its business day to day. So long as the pelvis is well placed, splits can lengthen and release the psoas (chronic tightness of which is a major cause of lower back pain and spasm, especially for the desk-bound), and when the pose is active (i.e. practised with muscles engaged rather than sinking to the floor) it can also lengthen and strengthen the hamstrings (gifting you the ability to tie your shoes) and stabilise the hips by strengthening the glutes (weakness of which can cause knee pain, and lower back, ankle, foot and shoulder problems).

Hanumanasana is also the door to a whole other room of yoga poses. Once you've conquered it the resulting strength and flexibility will make many of the postures in this book – especially the upside-down ones – a great deal easier.

What You Need:

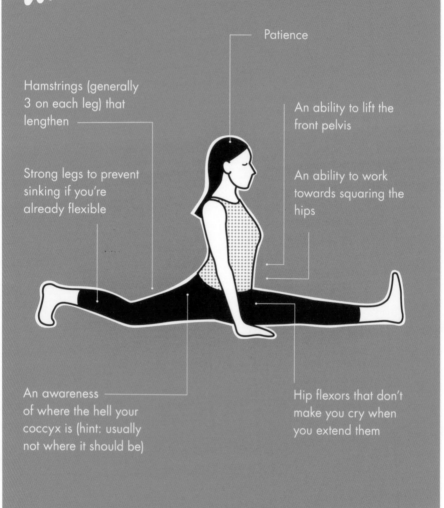

Patience

Hamstrings (generally 3 on each leg) that lengthen

An ability to lift the front pelvis

Strong legs to prevent sinking if you're already flexible

An ability to work towards squaring the hips

An awareness of where the hell your coccyx is (hint: usually not where it should be)

Hip flexors that don't make you cry when you extend them

Gateway Poses

The best way to work towards any pose is to practise a set of drills and 'gateway poses' that will help develop all of the important aspects, rather than trying to jam yourself into the posture from the get-go.

So practise the following regularly, and practise them honestly – if something hurts or you don't feel the work or the stretch in the right place, come out and try again. Listen to your body and only go as far as is sensible for you. Otherwise you're just hanging out in a weird shape for the good of nothing at all.

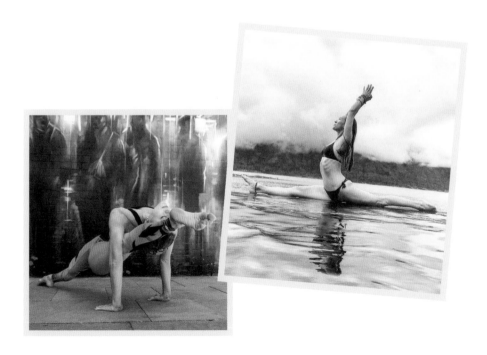

HIGH CRESCENT LUNGE

Similar to a Warrior 1 pose but with the back heel high, a lunge is a great place to practise your pelvic placement, and to start lengthening the deep hip flexors (the psoas).

Step into a lunge with the right leg forward, bending into the front leg with the back leg straight and the back heel off the ground. Look at your front leg and check your knee is no further forward than your front ankle, and the knee is not veering off to the left.

Now, to set your pelvis, bend the back leg and perform a small John-Travolta-style pelvic thrust, lifting the front points of your pelvis (ASIS) up and tucking the tailbone under. This action should give you a feeling of stretch in the hip flexors of your back leg. Once you feel this, re-straighten the back leg as much as you can, allowing the front points of the pelvis to drop a little, but keeping the stretch in the back leg, and not allowing your butt to stick out behind you. This control of the pelvis will be important in Hanumanasana.

Be careful not to let the front ribs stick out, as this usually means you've lost some control over the front body and core. Draw the lower ribs lightly towards one another but keep space to breathe, and if in doubt, make more space in the back of the ribs; this should automatically draw the front in. Keep your butt (the glutes) turned on and stretch the arms up overhead to lengthen the chest.

Stay here for 5 slow breaths (in for a count of 4, out for a count of 4). Work up to 10 breaths each side. To exit, step the feet back together and rest before taking the other side.

LOW DRAGON LUNGE

EQUIPMENT: Yoga bricks (optional)
SUBSTITUTION OPTIONS: Actual bricks/stacks of books/cans of beans

This is a very similar pose to the high lunge but (funnily enough) lower. It will get strongly into the psoas again, and if you're lucky, into the quads.

From your high lunge, place the hands on the floor or on yoga bricks either side of your front foot. If you're more flexible, take both hands to the floor inside your front foot.

You should already be feeling a stretch in the hip flexors of the back leg, but to intensify further, you can drop down to the elbows. The back knee can stay engaged and lifted so the back leg is straight, or you can drop down to the back knee, sinking the hips a little lower. Whichever way, keep your back toes tucked under and the back leg as active as you can. Also, make sure your front knee isn't winging out to the side; draw it in towards your shoulder.

Hold for 5 steady breaths, again working up to 10 on each side.

To exit, straighten the back leg if the knee was bending or dropped so you're back in a low runner lunge, push the hands into the ground (bring the hands to the ground first if the elbows were down) and step your front leg back to join the back one. Now you'll be in a plank. Drop to the knees, sit the butt to the heels and take the head to the floor with the arms outstretched. This is the Child's pose.

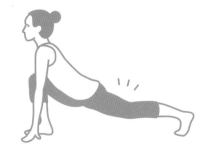

ANJANEYASANA

Low lunge with backbend (knees at right angles)

EQUIPMENT: A yoga blanket
SUBSTITUTION OPTIONS: A towel/an actual blanket/a small cushion

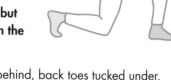

There are many versions of Anjaneyasana but this one will access the hip flexors and train the butt to keep working to aid stability.

Kneel, with right foot in front and left knee behind, back toes tucked under. Have right angles at both knee joints and try to keep it that way throughout.

Inhale and lift your arms high, stretch the chest upwards, squeeze the glutes and send the front hip points forwards and slightly up. Keep maximum space between your front thigh and the crest of your pelvis (ASIS), so they don't crunch together.

Hold and breathe. With each inhale lift the arms up and back towards the ears a little more, working the backbend in the upper spine. With each exhale send the hips forwards a little from the gluteal creases (where your butt becomes your leg). You should feel a deep stretch in the hip flexors of the back leg, and the sensation that you need to work incredibly hard with the butt to prevent yourself from sinking into the lower back.

If you feel a pinch in your lower back, come back up, reset the pelvis and try again. Keep the chin neutral and keep sending your heart upwards, without flaring the ribs.

Hold the pose for 5 steady breaths, working towards 10. To get out, inhale to lift the chest back to neutral (keeping the legs strong is key), take your front foot back, and come to a kneeling position, toes untucked. Repeat with the other leg in front.

SUPTA PADANGUSTHASANA A

Reclining big toe pose A

EQUIPMENT: A yoga strap
SUBSTITUTION OPTIONS: A belt (from your trousers)/a tie
(from your suit)/a scarf (from your under-stairs cupboard)

This is one for the hamstrings as well as for checking on pelvic placement and active legs.

Lie on your back with knees bent and feet on the floor. Bring your right knee into your chest. Take a yoga strap and loop it around the instep of the foot.

Hold each end of the strap, with enough slack to allow the elbows to draw towards the body and bend. Inhale and straighten out your right leg, foot towards the sky, and on an exhale do a little sit-up with the chest.

You can grab the toe with your right hand (if you have long arms), but a scarf or belt around your foot will also do nicely. Once you have a hold of your toe or strap, push your foot away from you. Use your core to maintain that small sit-up (so that just the tips of the shoulder blades are on the floor), and keep pulling with your arms. If you're flexible, don't bring the leg closer to you than a 12-o'clock angle – keep the foot pointing towards the sky. To intensify, straighten out your left leg along the floor, and press the back of your left thigh into the ground.

Hold for 5 breaths each leg, working up to 10. To release, slowly lower the right leg back to the ground. Then bend the knees up to your chest and give them a little hug towards the armpits to release the lower back, before taking the other side.

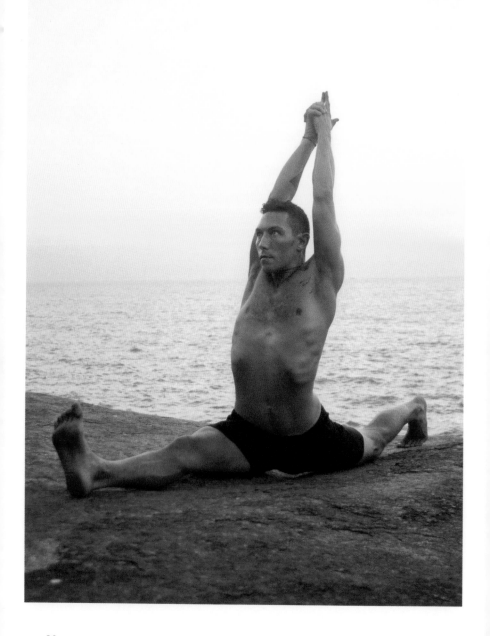

PADANGUSTHASANA

Standing forward fold/
Standing big toe pose

**This is another one for the hamstrings, as well as helping develop
an awareness of the angle of your hips and the direction of your
coccyx and sit bones.**

To begin, stand with your feet hip-width apart, inhale to lift your chest,
and on an exhale fold your body forwards. Bending the knees as much
as you need, take hold of your big toes with your peace fingers and
thumbs, then pull up on the toes as you push down with the feet.

For those with long noodles of hamstrings, work towards straightening
the legs by lifting the skin above the kneecaps upwards (making sure
your knees don't hyper-extend and 'lock' backward in the joints). For
those whose hamstrings are screaming at just the thought, keep bending
the knees as much as you need, making sure the knees don't knock in
towards one another. →

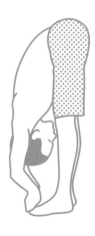

✴ IMPORTANT: If you are working with any hamstring injury, bending the knees in a forward fold is likely to be aggravating. Instead, keep the legs straight but bring the ground towards you by placing the hands on yoga blocks. Don't worry how little you fold: as long as you can feel a stretch in your hamstrings, you're in the right place.

Hold for 5 slow breaths, gradually working towards 10. Rather than twerking your sit bones up to the sky, draw the lower belly in and imagine you're folding over a small rolled-up towel placed at the hip crease. You don't want to be rounded and hunched like a tortoise, but you do want a small gap between the front hips and your thighs. This will allow the lumbar spine to stretch out.

To come out, release your grip on the toes, soften your knees, round your back and let the arms dangle for a few breaths, still folded forward, keeping the core (belly) lightly drawn in. When you're ready, roll up through the spine, keeping knees soft but butt engaged, all the way to standing.

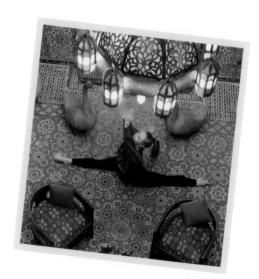

HALF HANUMANASANA A & B
Half splits

EQUIPMENT: Yoga bricks (optional)
SUBSTITUTION OPTIONS: Stacks of books/
boxes/actual bricks

**The final gateway pose is half
Hanumanasana. Here the hip flexors
don't get the same joyous stretch as in the
full thing, but the hamstrings get some extra fun instead.**

To begin, come to a low lunge position with the right leg in front. Drop your
back knee to the ground, and sit your butt back to your heel. Straighten out
the front leg and place the hands either on yoga bricks or on the floor, one
either side of your front leg. To intensify, walk the hands further away from
you towards your front ankle, perhaps even beyond the foot.

This is one version of the pose, and you can stay here – butt to heel, spine
long, either sitting upright or stretching forwards.

The second variation is to lift the butt off the back heel and stack the hips
directly above the back knee. Then from here, it's the same – stretch the
front heel forwards, and start to creep the fingertips towards the front of
the mat, or place the bricks under your hands if the floor seems a long
way away. How far forward you fold or how upright you sit will depend
on your hips, your hamstrings and the length of your arms. Do whatever
gives you a decent stretch in the back of the front leg without rounding or
hunching the shoulders.

In all options, keep the back toes tucked if you can.

Hold for 5 breaths each side, working up to 10. To exit, bend your front leg
and slide the foot towards you until you can place it on the floor. You can
stand up from here (or lie down and recover). Remember to do both sides.

Step by Step:

HOW TO HANUMANASANA

EQUIPMENT: Yoga bricks (optional), a yoga blanket (optional)
SUBSTITUTION OPTIONS: Books/boxes/actual bricks, towels/folded clothing

Once you've worked your hamstrings, your hip flexors and the strength of your legs, it's time to tackle the full pose.

Now, if you've had any ballet or gymnastic training, or if you simply have a conveniently roomy front pelvic crest, Hanumanasana may be a piece of vegan cake for you. For the rest of us it pays to take it slow, step by step.

1. Start out in a half Hanumanasana, with the back toes tucked, the front leg straight out in front, and the hands or fingertips resting on the floor or on bricks.

2. Pressing the hands lightly into the ground or the bricks, lift the chest and start to straighten out your back leg. Slowly. Once you come to the first significant point of resistance (i.e. your hamstrings and hip flexors are talking loudly to you), stop.

3. Hold at this point, with your legs engaged, and imagine you are drawing your legs towards each other so that the effect is to 'scissor' the hips – i.e. draw your back hip forwards and your front hip backwards.

4. Hold for 5 slow breaths.

5. If there's room to go deeper, allow your body to sink downwards slightly, keeping legs engaged, and hold for another 5 breaths.

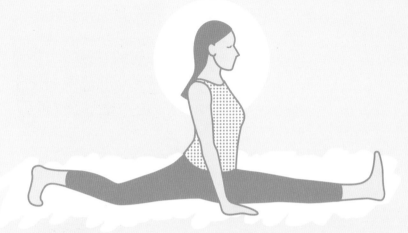

TO EXIT: push into the bricks or the floor with your hands and start to lift the pelvis higher, drawing the back leg in until the knee is back on the ground, and drawing the front foot in until you can place the sole of it back on solid earth. From here you can stand up or use furniture or a fellow human being to help you if your legs have turned to jelly.

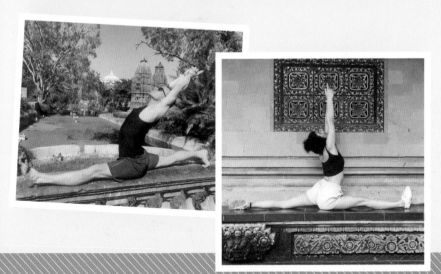

Hints & Tips

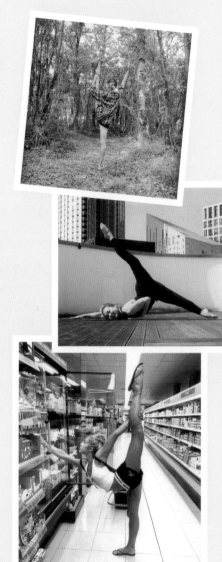

DO:

✳ Keep the back toes tucked under and push off the ball of the foot to activate the legs.

✳ Rotate your chest to be in line with the angle of your hips if you feel any discomfort in the lower back.

✳ Use bricks, blocks or books under your hands if you need them, so that you don't round the spine and hunch forwards.

✳ Place a towel or blanket under the back knee if it feels uncomfortable on the floor.

✳ Pay attention to the pelvis. Are you sticking your butt out like a Kardashian? If so, rein in the twerk. Try to lift the front hip points up and drop the back pelvis down. Check there is some space between your front thigh bone and the front of the pelvis (think of Padangusthasana pose).

DON'T:

* Hold the pose if you feel sharp pain (above all, make sure you can still breathe wherever you're holding).

* Just sink into your joints. If you're very flexible and you can get all the way to the floor, actively draw the legs towards one another so that the pelvis lifts an inch off the ground and hold it that way. Now you're working your muscles and gaining stability and strength around the joints.

* Hyper-extend your front knee. Be aware of the straight-leg knee locking backward. Put a brick or rolled-up towel under the front thigh if this is happening, then strongly lift the muscles above the kneecap upwards.

* Stick the ribs out in front of you. Lifting the front hips up should help draw them back, but so will lightly drawing the ribs closed (without constricting your breathing).

TAKING IT TO THE NEXT LEVEL

Once you're snugly in your splits, you can play with the arms and the legs. You can reach the arms high to stretch the chest and increase the work in your legs; you can bend up your back leg and hook the same elbow around it, stretching your hip flexors and quads and introducing an element of a backbend; or you can take a splits to standing with the hands on bricks or the floor (which becomes a case of balancing well on your grounded foot), or even standing without touching the floor at all (which becomes just a case of serious balance).

#Instatips

Once you're in Hanumanasana, there is a plethora of variations to play with. You can sit, stand, lift the arms to the sky, take a fold forward, bend up the back leg or lift up the front one. The choices are endless.

LOCATION, LOCATION, LOCATION

For your basic seated, straight-legged Hanumanasana, the composition of the photo is everything. It is best performed on some sort of ledge, whether that's a sun lounger on the beach or those invisible walls built into exotic swimming pools, presumably for just this sort of photo opportunity.

For an urban shot, get experimental. Remember: all furniture, architecture and machinery is at your disposal – closing lift doors at work present an excellent opportunity to both irritate Carol who is trying to get

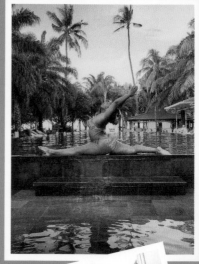

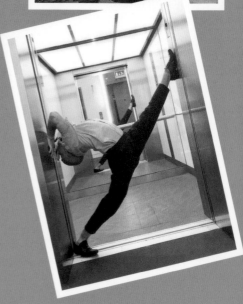

to the meeting on the fourth floor and to show off your legs, and the frozen-food aisle can only be enhanced with one of your feet sticking up in the air.

COSTUME

In general, the fewer clothes the better, but in this pose especially, avoid anything baggy that might mask the long line of your legs. For swimming pool or wall shots, a bikini, tiny shorts or trunks are obligatory. Good hair is a must, ideally flowing in a light breeze.

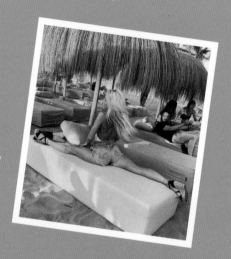

PROPS

The standing variation of this pose is most effective in nature. Choose a dense forest where the lines of your arms and legs can mimic nature's patterns, or wooden fences in rural environments where you can hang or dangle in an interesting way.

If you actually require props (like a yoga brick for the hands), don't let the idea of 'yoga' limit your choices – choose interesting objects, such as a pair of trainers, to act as your aids.

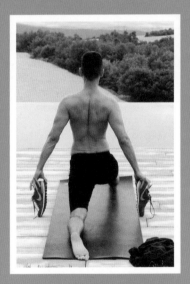

DANGER RATING

7/10

Hanumanasana scores fairly low on the SAS (Suicidal Asana Scale) in terms of risk of sudden or severe falls, but the chance of requiring replacement of body parts is high. For the stiffer yogi, there is a chance of muscle strain in the hips or hamstrings, which would register as a 3 out of 10. However, for the hyper-mobile Instayogi (whose super-splits are part of their gentle morning stretch) the chance of gradual labrum tear and eventual hip replacement if not performed actively and with care is high, taking Hanumanasna up to a hip-splitting 7.

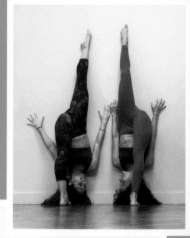

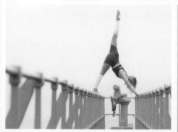

EXIT STRATEGY

There is little danger of falling out of a seated splits, as floor is one of the hardest things to fall off. If you choose to try the splits on a wall, try to ensure a grassy verge, a bush or a friend may be able to catch you.

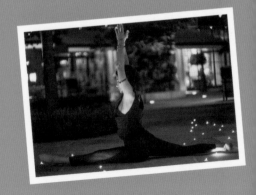

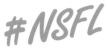

(NOT SAFE FOR LIFE)

Here we travel to the very edges of creative Instagramming, as true art walks a thin line between greatness and craziness. This is our friend Wen.

She tried to demonstrate Pythagoras's theorem and ended up collapsing space and time. Sometimes it is possible to go too far. Sometimes it is possible to be too flexible. That time is here. #broken

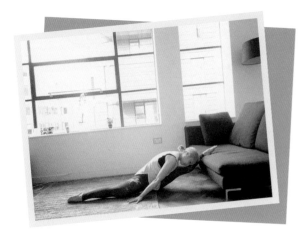

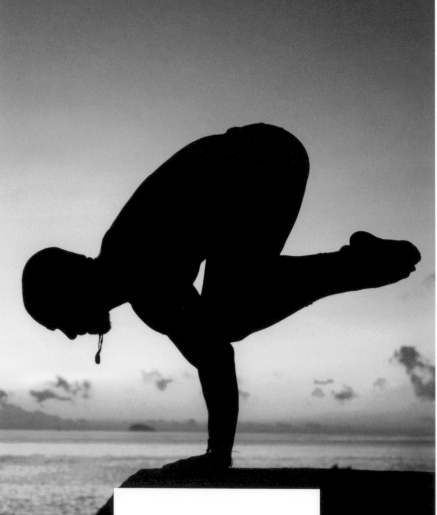

BAKASANA

2

Crow pose

Bakasana, or Crow pose, also has a bundle of variations. It can be performed with straight or bent elbows, with feet together or one leg extended, and it can be a transitional pose towards casually pressing to a handstand or dropping slowly to a headstand.

As well as being an Instagram favourite, Bakasana also has an array of physical benefits. It stabilises the scapulae (shoulder blades) and back, strengthens the arms and the wrists, and develops wrist flexion and hip mobility. Importantly, it also teaches you to face the abyss (in this case the hard floor in front of your face) without fear, or at least to work slowly towards staring into it.

What You Need:

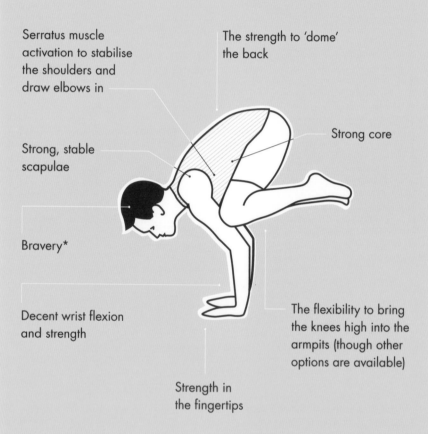

Serratus muscle activation to stabilise the shoulders and draw elbows in

The strength to 'dome' the back

Strong core

Strong, stable scapulae

Bravery*

Decent wrist flexion and strength

The flexibility to bring the knees high into the armpits (though other options are available)

Strength in the fingertips

*or a pillow on the floor in front of your face

Gateway Poses

If done correctly these gateway poses will build strength and positioning for a Bakasana of dreams.

WRIST STRETCHES

Full Bakasana calls for a fairly intense load on flexed wrists, so start by warming up and working the range of motion in the wrists. (Although the pose can be modified to suit tighter wrists, it definitely should not be attempted with a wrist injury.)

Come to all fours, wrists under the shoulders and knees under the hips, fingers spread wide. Shift weight from right hand to left hand, eventually leaning the body as far to the right and the left as is comfortable. Repeat, shifting forwards and backwards over the wrists, eventually moving the body in slow circles all around the wrists first one way and then the other.

The second stretch is a little more intense, so go slow. Sit the butt back to the heels so that you're kneeling. Turn the palms up to the sky. Sit up a little off your heels and slowly place the fingertips on the floor, palms now facing away from you. With the fingertips pointing towards you, place the rest of the fingers on the ground, then the palms of the hands, eventually stretching all the way to the wrist so that the whole hand is on the floor.

By moving into an all-fours position, hips over knees, this stretch is less intense. Taking the butt back towards the heels will make it more intense. Remember to go slow, and never work through any sharp pain.

Finally, repeat the stretch above but reverse the palms. The fingers still face towards you, but the backs of the hands slowly lower to the floor.

It's sometimes nice to start this one on all fours again (be careful not to take too much weight into the hands) and then slowly start to sit back towards the heels (not necessarily all the way) to deepen the stretch.

Take these stretches slow, and work into them gradually, taking a minute or two over each one. Once you're done, give the wrists a good shake out.

GYMNASTIC PLANK

This exercise gets right to the core (which will help lift your hips high in the pose) as well as nailing the position of the back – primarily the sensation of pushing the hands into the ground while protracting (separating) the shoulder blades, which is an essential part of a stable Bakasana.

The gymnastic plank differs from the more common Pilates-style plank by emphasising a 'domed' upper back, drawing the inner borders of the shoulder blades apart and the bottom tips of them into the back, making a visible curve of the upper spine. This is one of the major actions you need in a Crow.

Start on all fours. Check the hands are directly beneath the shoulders and the joints of the fingers are firmly grounded. Push the base of the thumbs and index fingers into the ground. Spin the bones of the tops of the arms outward in external rotation (your arms are unlikely to spin out that visibly, but it's the muscle action of the rotation that is important) and think of drawing the inner elbows towards one another. It can help to enlist a friend to place a hand on your upper back, which you can push to the sky in order to feel the doming action.

When the arms are in place, tuck your toes and lift your knees off the ground to a plank, stretching the heel bones back. Draw the belly button lightly to the spine, engage the glutes and push the hands into the floor, protracting the shoulder blades, sending them wrapping under your arms while the space between them rises to the sky.

Try to hold for 10 breaths. Watch out for the pelvis, which often has a life of its own. It will either want to droop down (therefore pinching into your lower back) or lift up (taking you halfway to a Down Dog). Think instead of drawing the bones at the front of your pelvis towards your ribs, so the lower back stays long.

To exit, drop the knees to the floor, sit the butt to the heels and take a Child's pose.

HALF CHATURANGA DANDASANA
(elbows bent & knees on the floor)

The knees-down Chaturanga variation is often seen as the less-cool sibling of full Chaturanga, yet when it is done well, it is an enormous shoulder and serratus strengthener, stabiliser and body placement aid. More to the point, it is a considerably more useful pose than the shaking, sweating, poorly executed full Chaturanga that so many people seem bent on performing 105 times per class.

Begin in your domed/gymnastic plank with elbows stacked over wrists. On an inhale, slightly shift to the tips of your toes so that your whole body shifts forwards and, depending on your range of motion at the wrists, you may have your shoulders over the mid-hand. On an exhale drop to your knees, keeping your pelvis slightly tucked so you are in a half-plank position. Slowly bend the elbows, hugging the elbows in towards the ribs and stacking your elbow joints directly over your wrists, keeping the belly in and the glutes on. The core should be engaged (no butt tilts, hikes or droops) and you are aiming for a 90-degree angle at each elbow to avoid strain on the ligaments.

Once you're in, hold for 5 steady breaths, then lower the whole body to the floor, lie on your belly and rest. Repeat, eventually working up to 5 rounds.

NB It can be hard to tell where 90 degrees is at the elbow. You can try this alongside a mirror, or film yourself (for your own benefit, not for Insta) in order to see how acute or open the elbows are.

FULL CHATURANGA

For the full whammy, again start in your domed plank and on an inhale shift to the tips of the toes. This time keep the kneecaps lifting so the legs stay straight (and the heels stretch back, just like plank pose) as you slowly bend the elbows to 90 degrees. Core is on, front hips are slightly lifted towards the ribs to avoid twerking, drooping or tilting the pelvis, and legs and glutes are on to keep the butt firm.

Keep hugging the elbows towards your ribs and squeeze the shoulder blades towards each other. Your body should still be in one long line, just with the elbows bending.

Hold for 5 breaths, then either continue your Vinyasa – coming into Up Dog then Down Dog and hold for a few breaths before the next round – or drop the knees to the floor as before and bring yourself all the way to the ground and rest. Take 3 to 5 rounds.

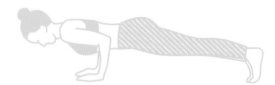

HALF CROW
(knees by the elbows)

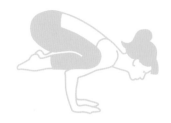

EQUIPMENT: You might want a pillow
under your delicate face
SUBSTITUTION OPTIONS: Cushions/blankets/folded-up clothing

If you feel ready to try Crow but you want to ease yourself in, start with a half Crow. Whereas the full Crow has the knees high towards the armpits and you are working your arms towards being straight, half Crow has bent elbows (possibly even 90 degrees) with the knees resting just above the elbow joint. The result is a much flatter shape of the body, with your chest a little lower to the ground and parallel to the floor. This gives you the opportunity to practise the balance of weight in the arms without the peril of having so far to fall.

Start crouched on the floor and place your hands on the ground, shoulder-width apart. Ground the joints of the fingers and start to lean the body forward, coming to your tiptoes and bending the elbows until you can place the knees on the upper arms just above the elbow joint.

From here, it is all about counterbalance, so start to tip the body forward until the feet become lighter and lighter, and the chest gradually becomes parallel to the ground. If you feel comfortable, lift one or maybe both feet just an inch off the ground. If you're worried about face-planting, position a pillow on the floor in front of you for a soft landing.

If you find flight, hold for 5 slow breaths. To exit, bring the feet (not your face) to the floor, lower the knees down and rest in Child's pose.

Step by Step:

HOW TO BAKASANA

EQUIPMENT: You might again want your trusty face pillow

Once you've found that elusive counterbalance in half Crow, and can hold your various Chaturangas and planks with some stability (and less furious shaking), you'll be ready to try the full pose.

1. From a standing position, fold forward, place your hands on the floor, and start to bend your knees towards your armpits, coming to your tiptoes as you do.

2. Press the joints of the index fingers and the thumbs down, and spin the tops of the arms open (external rotation of the humerus bones), like in plank pose.

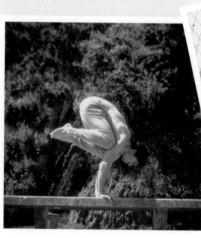

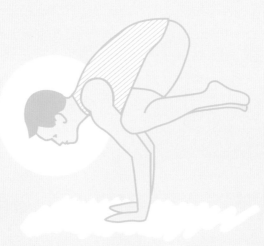

3. Dome your back, draw in your core, and start to tip the weight into the arms, becoming lighter on the feet.

4. If you feel balanced, lift one foot off the floor. Hold and stabilise by pushing hands down and drawing the elbows towards each other. Repeat with the other foot. If you feel ready, lift both feet off the floor, bring the toes together and squeeze the heels towards your butt. Breathe!

5. If you feel comfortable and can hold steadily for 5 breaths, work towards straightening the arms and making the knees lighter against the armpits.

TO EXIT: bring your feet back to earth and rest.

DO:

* Place a pillow or blanket in front of you if you're worried about falling on your face.

* Hug the inner elbows towards one another.

* Hug the knees inward rather than letting them slide outward of the arms.

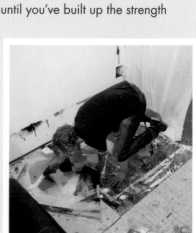

* Look up a little as you lean into the balance – your head will help to counterbalance your butt (but don't look up so far that you strain your neck).

* Keep the arms as bent as you need to until you've built up the strength in the arms, back and core to straighten them a little.

* Start with the knees lower down the arm to begin with if that feels less frightening for you, and gradually work the knees towards being in the armpits as you feel more confident.

* Persevere! Crow pose is a mixture of very specific strength, flexibility and understanding the counterbalance of your body. Take your time and keep trying.

DON'T:

* Drop your head to stare at the floor. This usually results in a forward roll or eating the carpet.

* Allow the weight to sway significantly to the outside of the hands. This tends to overload the outer wrist and can lead to wrist aches, pains and strains.

* Continue to practise if your wrists start hurting.

* Jump. Always lift slowly off the feet by pushing into the hands and tipping, coming right to the tiptoes before lift-off to begin with.

* Try to straighten the arms before you're ready – and only do so if you have been dealt flexible wrists in the joint-mobility lottery. This variation requires the shoulders moving forwards towards the fingers, creating an acute angle at the wrist joint, so make sure you have a safe range of motion to try.

TAKING IT TO THE NEXT LEVEL

Once you have the Crow shape down, you can start to have fun with the legs. Perhaps try Eka Pada Bakasana, one-legged Crow pose (though this requires great stability of the shoulders, so is not for those new to the Crow flight). For this one, once you're in Crow, lean the chest forward, push the ground away, and start to shift the majority of the weight into your left knee rather than sharing it between the two. If the right knee becomes light you can start to lift it off the back of your arm. If all is going well and you're not yet in a heap, start to straighten the right leg up and back. Keep the chest stretching forward to counterbalance the back leg extending. Remember learning about levers in physics at school? Turns out it was useful after all.

#Instatips

The bit you've been waiting for: it's time to take another picture. Remember, unlike actual yoga, you do not need to hold an Instagram posture in a stable or enduring way, and you don't even need to breathe properly (unless you have your camera on a long timer and have to wait for it to flash).

LOCATION, LOCATION, LOCATION

Height is your friend for the Crow. Consider a rock (best of all, one with a sudden drop or a seascape behind you), a high ledge, wall or bench, and ideally with a feature of interest or an urban landmark behind you. Wherever you are, try to take the picture from the side, since this is how you will give the most impressive sense of flying. As with the majority of Instapics, sunset or sunrise are both excellent choices, but Bakasana is especially effective in silhouette.

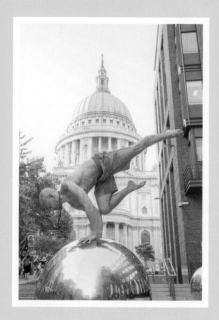

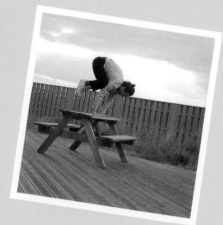

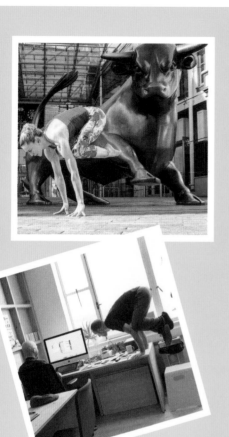

COSTUME

For Crow pose, being able to see your legs is a bonus. Consider a bikini, mini shorts or the male legging (the 'megging').

It's important to note that although a deeply moisturised and glowing body is a vital element of your Insta photography, slippery knees and arms do not make for successful Bakasanas. If you must douse yourself in shine spray, make sure your knees or pits are covered so you can grip without sliding to the floor.

PROPS

For the male yogi, a beard goes down a treat. Consider investing in a prop beard if you are unwilling or unable to grow your own. Beards lend gravitas. They also catch the light well.

Also, try performing this pose with adorable children, especially babies, especially directly beneath your precariously balanced face. Looming over the young is cute but also lends an element of jeopardy, which can only translate into Likes.

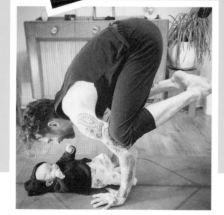

DANGER RATING

Bakasana has a fairly high rating due to its danger-to-face factor (which of course has implications for future Instagram pictures), bringing it in at a solid 7, though this can be lowered by placing pillows, cushions or crash mats on the floor in front of you (out of sight of the camera ideally, or they can always be Photoshopped out later). Similarly, you might choose to perform the asana on soft ground, such as sand or grass. The Suicidal Asana rating can be raised to a 9 or 10 if performing this arm balance on uneven rocks, where it is difficult to ensure a good hand grip, or on precarious ledges, where the chance of falling to severe injury or even death is high.

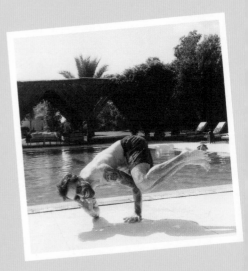

EXIT STRATEGY

If you are on low and soft ground and you cannot bring the weight back to the feet, the best emergency exit from Bakasana is a chin-tuck forward roll. If performed at height, there is no safe way to emergency-exit this pose.

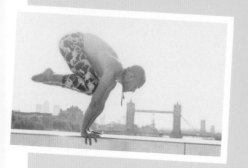

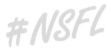

(NOT SAFE FOR LIFE)

Out of a desire to be inclusive and show #atmos, you might be tempted to involve extras in your picture. Do not over-populate and, above all, do not engage Instayoga novices (with the obvious exception of babies and dogs).

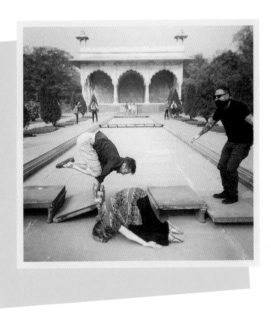

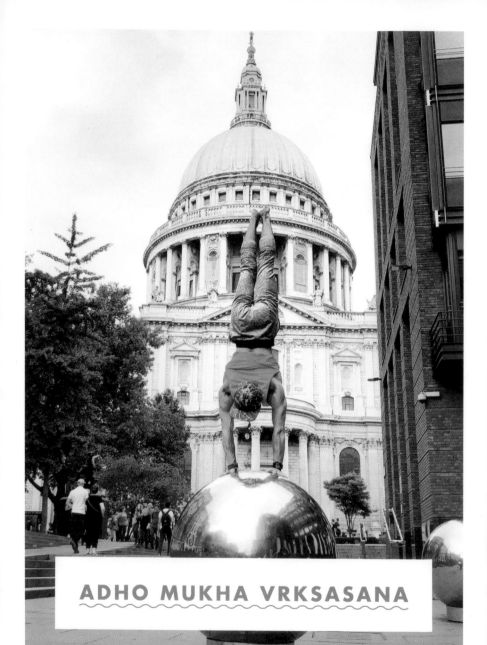

ADHO MUKHA VRKSASANA

3

Handstand

As well as being the pose that wins you all the prizes at parties, a handstand – both working towards one and doing one – can bring about big changes in the body and the mind. For people without a background in Olympic gymnastics, they take enormous patience, tenacity and focus, which are skills many of us need to develop. They also ask an enormous amount of the body and your awareness of it.

Secondly, the precise balance to stay in a handstand requires activation of stabilising muscles in everything from the fingertips to the toes, engaging every finger, lengthening the spine and stabilising the shoulders while being able to make micro-shifts in each of these things in order to save the balance if you start to tip. Thirdly, finding even a moment of perfect balance can bring a brief but total stillness of the mind. The moment you start to think in a handstand is the moment you immediately flop out of your handstand.

Handstands can be performed in many ways with many leg and arm variations, but there are two distinct forms with the hands – often referred to as 'yoga' handstands and 'gymnastic' handstands. The former has arms a little wider apart (which is easier to transition to and from during Vinyasa (flowing) sequences), and the latter has the hands very narrow. We will look at drills and options for both.

Both are mega hits on Instagram.

What You Need:

Back strength

Core strength to keep a bendy back in line

Decent range of motion at the shoulder joint (some versions require the arms alongside the ears)

Stable shoulders and scapulae (shoulder blades)

The calmness to resist furiously hurling yourself into the air before you have control

Decent wrist strength and flexion

The bravery to try

Gateway Poses

More than for any other, the gateway poses for a handstand really do need to be stable before you start flinging your legs into the air like you just don't care without a wall or someone to spot you. The following exercises are a mix of stability, strengthening and range of motion.

WRIST & HAMSTRING EXERCISES

Before you begin a handstand practice session, it's important to make sure the wrists are warm and at your best range of motion. You will be taking a lot of weight into them while they are flexed. We've covered these bad boys in the section on Bakasana, so run through some or all of those exercises.

Similarly, long hamstrings will be an enormous advantage for stepping into your handstand, as they will enable you to get one leg high in the sky, meaning the hips are higher and less pushing off the grounded foot is needed. Having to push less means more control as you come up, and less likelihood of bombing out the other side. So also practise the hamstring stretches in the Hanumanasana section, as well as Hanumanasana itself.

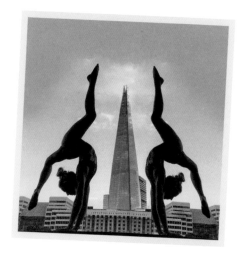

SUPINE DISH ABS

The most fun of all the ab exercises. This one trains the shape of your handstand (any inversion, in fact) by working the core and reining in the butt twerk (especially important for the bendy banana-backed among you).

Start by lying on your back on a mat so your spine doesn't crunch into the floor. Take your hands behind your head and cup the base of the skull and neck. You can keep the elbows wide or, if the neck feels strained, draw the elbows in so that you've made a full support for the head.

Bend your knees and bring the knees over the hips so the shins are flat like a table. Now inhale and roll your upper body up so that only the bottom tips of your shoulder blades remain on the floor. Exhale and straighten your legs, lowering them as much as you can towards the floor without your lower back leaving the ground. If you are naturally lordotic (i.e. you have a naturally arched back), your legs may not lower very far before this happens. If this is the case, keep the legs as high as they need to be to keep the back down. Inhale and return the legs to tabletop position.

Repeat this straightening and bending 10 times. On the final one, hold the legs in the outstretched position and count to 5 (working up eventually to 10), then bend the knees in to the chest, release the head and shoulders down, and relax.

This is a pretty tough exercise if you do it correctly, but should you want to make it even harder, as you extend and lower the legs, stretch the arms back over your head, then return them to the head as you bend the knees back in. Enjoy.

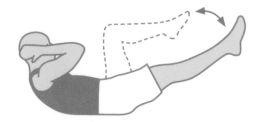

TURBO FLYING PLANK

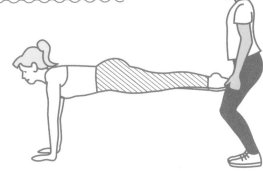

EQUIPMENT: A friend
SUBSTITUTION OPTIONS:
A friendly looking stranger
with little else to do with
their day

**You are by now intimately
familiar with the domed
plank, which can very much
count as one of your handstand drills. To take it up a level and make it
more handstand-specific, you can also practise the turbo flying plank.
For this, you will need to rope in a friend as a willing foot-holder.**

Start in your domed-back plank, pushing the ground away, controlling
the line of the pelvis. Now ask your recruited foot-friend to lift your legs
off the ground, holding one ankle in each of their hands, until your feet
reach the height of your shoulders. Keep squeezing your legs together
and slightly tuck the tailbone. You should look like one long line from your
head to your toes.

Now, keeping the belly in, the glutes on and your legs squeezing
together, ask your friend to let go of one of your ankles. Ideally, don't
let them tell you which one. It adds to the excitement. Once the ankle is
released, do not let it drop even an inch. Hold for 1 or 2 breaths, then
beg your friend to take hold of your ankle again.

Repeat this on different ankles.

Aim for 10 ankle-drops, then your friend can lower your feet back to
the ground, and you can lie down, take a Child's pose, or curl up in a
ball to recover.

HANDSTAND AGAINST A WALL

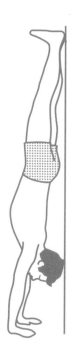

Once you've found a stable plank, turbo flying plank and you've got your head around the dish abs shape, you can try using a wall to handstand.

Place the hands on the ground a foot away from the wall. Root down through the finger joints and the tips of the fingers, spin the elbow creases forward and look between your hands. Walk in as close to your hands as your hips and hamstrings will let you and stick one leg up to the sky. This top leg is your guide – so engage it, lengthen it and point the toe skywards.

Now, without hurling yourself into the air, soften the leg on the ground and push off it – a small jump at first, squeezing the butt cheek of the flying leg and pointing the top foot to the sky. Do this a few times, focussing on the top leg and imagining that is what is pulling you up.

When you feel ready, see if you can reach the top leg towards the wall and bring your bottom leg up to join it. This may take a few attempts, but each time push down into the floor with the hands like you're pushing it away, activate the top leg, and once the bottom leg has left the floor keep it light or it will pull you back down.

Once you get both legs up, rest the heels against the wall and stretch them towards the sky. This should lengthen the back of the pelvis and help take out any over-arching of the back. Keep pushing the hands into the ground, keep the elbows straight and stack them over the wrists as much as you can. Keep the legs on (which is usually the bit people forget) and keep the core engaged.

Once you start to feel confident, perhaps take one foot an inch away from the wall, and then maybe the other one joins it. Hold, to begin with, for 5 breaths (feet on or off the wall). Work up to 10 breaths to build stamina.

To come out, bring one leg down to the floor at a time and then repeat the handstand, this time pushing off the other leg.

This can be performed with either hand position – hands a little wider than the shoulders (yoga handstand), or in line with or narrower than the shoulders (gymnastic handstand).

PIKE OR 'L' HANDSTAND ON A WALL

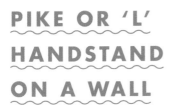

Once you have the confidence and stamina to hold a steady handstand with your back to the wall, it's time to turn to face it. The pike or 'L' position, with hands on the floor and feet on the wall, is more demanding on the shoulders and core, and helps you practise stacking the hips over the shoulders, keeping the pelvis in line.

Start by sitting on the floor with your back against the wall and legs stretched out in front of you and take note of the position of your feet. When you stand up, you want to put your hands where your feet were, so that they're a leg length away from the wall.

Once the hands are in the required position, start to walk your feet up the wall until they are in line with your hips, then bend your knees a little – this is your rest position. →

From here, push the hands to the ground and the feet to the wall and straighten the legs. You should now be in an upside-down 'L' shape. The position of your hands is key – if your hands are too far from the wall, your body will be sloping and the shoulders not stacked over the wrists. If your hands are too close to the wall, your back will arch and your hips (and butt) will stick out beyond the line of your wrists.

Once you find that Goldilocks position, push the ground away and hold for 10 seconds, working up to 30 seconds (which is hard).

The progression of this pose, once you can hold it steadily for 30 seconds, is to lift one leg straight to the sky, while the other one stays on the wall. Go slow and be careful with the top leg – if you overshoot, you're going over . . . Once you're stable on both legs (and can hold for 30 seconds), you can play with very, very slowly lifting the foot off the wall behind you. Then you will be in a free-standing handstand, with legs split at 90 degrees.

NB It is usually a good idea to have a friend on hand to 'spot' you (i.e. catch you) in this one-leg variation, as it's difficult to make a graceful dismount if you tip too far.

To come out of any of these variations, just walk the feet back down the wall to the ground – you can walk the hands away from the wall a little to give you more space too.

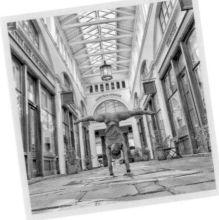

ZOMBIE
PRESS

EQUIPMENT: A pair of socks
SUBSTITUTION OPTIONS: A teatowel/
a bath towel/an item of clothing

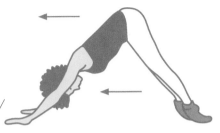

This exercise builds back strength and core while also cleaning your floors. It also helps build towards the elusive 'press' (rather than jump) into handstand.

You will need a smooth surface, such as tiles or floorboards (and you should travel in the direction of the boards if possible), and a small towel/ cloth or a pair of socks. Wear the socks, or place your bare feet on a small towel or cloth on the floor. You will also need the length of a room to travel.

Start in a plank, but with your toes pointed and the tops of the feet resting on your towel (or the floor if in socks). Inhale, and on the exhale push the hands into the ground, dome your back, draw the belly in and drag your feet along the floor towards your hands. Get as close to the hands as you can, right up on tiptoes, then flip the feet so the soles of the feet land lightly on the floor. Walk the hands out forwards to a plank again, point the toes with the tops of the feet on the floor and repeat. Travel across the room this way.

Try to get in 5 repetitions at least (even if you have to change direction and come back the other way). Work up to 10. If you're feeling energetic, then 20.

Once you get stronger, when the feet are right on tiptoes next to your hands, you may be able to hover the feet off the floor in order to flip them and return the soles of the feet to the ground. This, however, takes a lot of strength and a lot of hamstring and wrist flexibility, so it will take a long time to get there. The first exercise is strong enough!

Step by Step:

HOW TO HANDSTAND

Once you can perform these drills with stability and manage to hold them – in a good alignment – for a good 20–30 seconds, you're ready to leave the safety of the wall.

For the free-standing handstand, you might again want to enlist someone to spot you for the first few times. Not only will it save your vegan bacon if you fall, but it can encourage you to push a little harder and lift a little further to find the balance point, which is always an inch further away than feels 'safe'.

1. Find a space where you are not likely to destroy furniture. Grassy parks and gardens are especially good for soft handstand falls (and damage limitation). Fold forward and place your hands on the ground. Spread the fingers, ground the fingertips and walk your feet towards them as far as you can.

2. Lift your favourite leg to the sky. Point it strongly and engage the butt cheek attached to it.

3. Soften the supporting leg, tip your weight forwards into your hands – ideally get the shoulders over the wrists, if not further forward – and look in between your thumbs.

4. Take a small push off your grounded foot (try not to leap). As soon as you leave the ground push extra hard into your hands and point furiously

through your top leg. Try not to over-tense the bottom one. At first work on just finding a moment of hover before the foot comes back down.

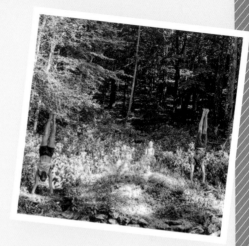

5. As you become more confident, the time between take-off and landing will become longer and your hips will be lifting higher. Once you find the glorious balance keep the legs split for a while – like with the wall exercise – as you can use them to counterbalance. Only when you can hold for a good 20 seconds in a split-leg position should you start to bring the lower leg up to join the top one for your legs-together handstand. Once you arrive, squeeze the legs together.

TO EXIT: ideally bring the legs back down the way you came. Other exit options include cartwheeling out, where you take one hand away from the floor and allow the legs to cartwheel to the ground in the direction of the hand you removed (turning cartwheels in a row is a great exercise to practise for falling out), or – controversially – landing in a full Wheel pose (a backbend) if you tip over. The backbend option is not a good idea for handstand beginners unless you have a lot of control (and sufficient flexibility), and even then it tends to encourage over-arching the back.

The final option is to step one hand forwards if you feel you are tipping too far one way, which will help bring your weight back so that you can bring your feet to the floor safely.

Hints & Tips

DO:

* Get someone to spot you if you need it while you're getting used to the balance and to falling out of the pose safely.

* Push down firmly into the ground every time you leave the ground.

* Get strong in the fingertips so you can use them to control your balance. If you tip slightly too far, it's your fingertips that will bring you back to centre.

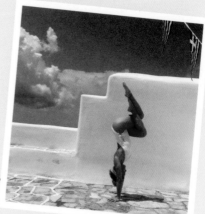

* Use your top leg, especially the glutes, to stab the sky and pull you up.

* Keep the legs split so you can control your balance with their counterweight.

TAKING IT TO THE NEXT LEVEL

Make sure you are super solid in your hand balancing before you start to mess with the legs, but once you are ready, you can start to work towards taking legs wide to the sides (in a 'straddle' handstand) or wrapping the legs around one another in the air. You can also take it back to the '80s and do Running Man legs in the air, bending at the knees, as though you got stuck mid-run, and holding it there.

DON'T:

* Sway your weight to just one part of the wrist or hand – there will be moments you will need to press into one area more than another if you are losing the balance in order to correct yourself, but be aware if you're developing a habit of sitting back in the wrists in particular. (Most commonly, your weight will fall to the heels of the wrists or the outsides of the wrists. If this tends to be a problem for you, practise your hand position and weight distribution kneeling on all fours: this will help develop good habits.)

* Tense the leg you're pushing off too strongly; try to make it light otherwise it most likely will pull you back to the ground.

* Arch your back and stick out your butt. If you're a bendy-back person you need extra core strength to stop yourself flopping out into a backbend on the other side.

* Kick wildly. Step in as close as you can (which will depend largely on your hamstrings) and push rather than leap off your bottom leg. You need a great deal of shoulder stability to stop the trajectory if you launch off too strongly without the control to stop at the top.

* Overuse your neck. It's actually a nice practice to try kicking up with your neck long, looking to the foot you're kicking off. Scary as hell – because you can't see where you're kicking to – but it will help to stop you tensing the muscles of the neck to pull you up. At the least, try to look at the space in between your thumbs rather than in front of your hands if your neck starts to pull.

#Instatips

The great thing about handstands is that there are so many options for looking mega skilful, even without actually being able to do a handstand.

LOCATION, LOCATION, LOCATION

If you can actually do a handstand, it can be performed to great effect almost anywhere, but they are especially impressive in an environment in which your pose is clearly impeding the ability of other people to go about their day.

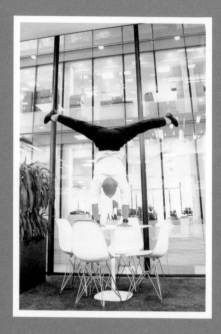

For instance, try at your desk at work while Carol is now trying to write up her minutes. Consider important architectural bridges at lunch hour, busy city-centre tourist attractions or public post boxes. If you can stay motionless for a while as others buzz around you, this also makes an important point about the superiority of your stillness in a world full of inferior moving people.

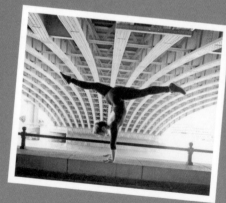

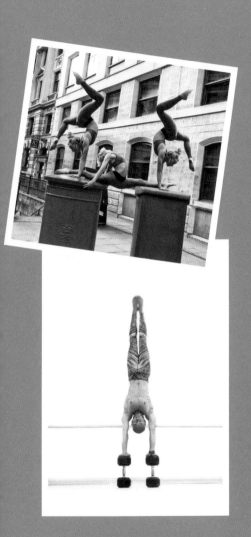

COSTUME

For the full 'just busted this out of nowhere' vibe, look like a civilian – the less practical your outfit, the better. Dress in a suit if you're at work (trouser or loose skirt), or the usual bikini, Lycra or catsuit if elsewhere, just as long as you are deeply tanned (from a bottle if necessary). Whatever you're wearing must allow you the stretch to get in and out of the handstand, but the restrictiveness of the costume or how revealing it is don't really matter. Don't think of it as a potential wardrobe danger, think of it as an opportunity.

PROPS

As always monuments, gym equipment and giant ball bearings (see picture on p. 48) up the artistic ante. As do other people also doing handstands, especially in nature.

For the holiday genre, think handstands on golden beaches, on rocks or on Grecian walkways. Be sure to coordinate your outfit with the colours of the town or landscape around you.

DANGER RATING

The SAS of a handstand can vary greatly. Handstanding at work has the risk of loss of gainful employment, and therefore loss of ability to pay for more handstand and yoga classes, which scores it around a 5 on the SAS scale (because what life is worth living without a handstand guru?). Adding height or indeed taking away width can raise the score. Handstanding on a narrow wall or ledge can take things up to an 8, and easily to a 9 if combined with height.

Handstanding in public also holds potential for collateral damage, taking the rating – when all lives and limbs are considered – to a solid 7.

EXIT STRATEGY

A full-on crash mat is the ideal scenario. But if one is not immediately available in an office environment, ask a colleague to catch you, or exit with a cartwheel if you have the balls.

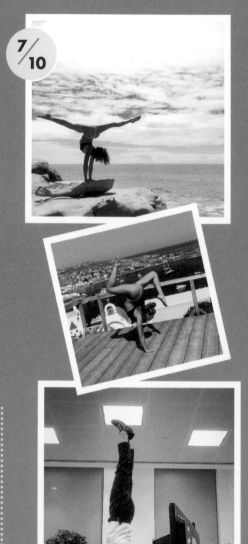

7/10

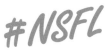

#NSFL

(NOT SAFE FOR LIFE)

Although scenery is important, do not allow it to overtake your pose. You are the centre of this Insta-universe: make sure your handstand is visible in all its glory.

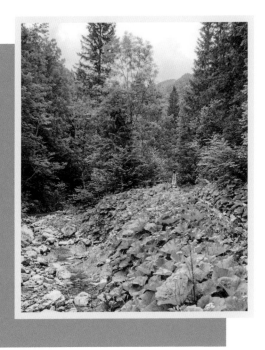

ASHTAVAKRASANA

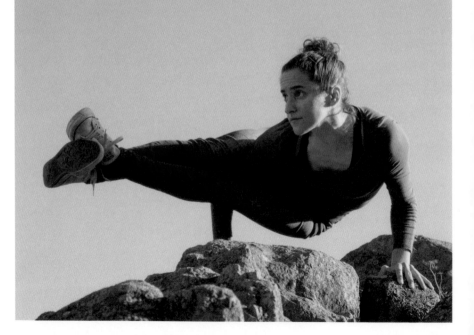

4

Crazy 8 pose

Ashtavakrasana or Crazy 8 pose is one of the obligatory funky arm balances. Named after a sage whose body was bent in 8 places as a result of his father mispronouncing his Vedic verses (long story...), the pose strengthens the shoulders, promotes stability around the shoulder blades and seriously engages the core. What's more, it teaches you to counterbalance your head and your butt. Which is what life is all about.

What You Need:

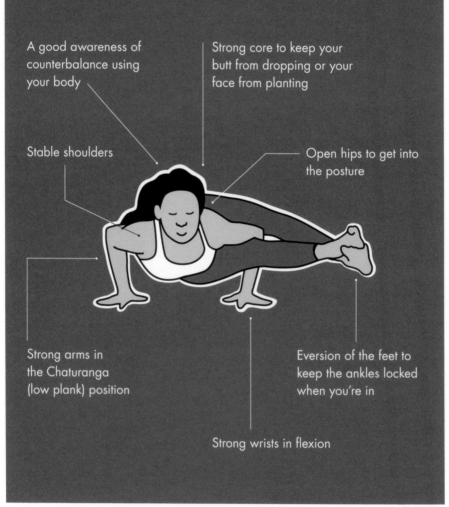

A good awareness of counterbalance using your body

Strong core to keep your butt from dropping or your face from planting

Stable shoulders

Open hips to get into the posture

Strong arms in the Chaturanga (low plank) position

Eversion of the feet to keep the ankles locked when you're in

Strong wrists in flexion

Gateway Poses

As an arm balance, just like Bakasana (Crow) and handstand, it's a good idea to start your warm-up with wrist stretches, planks and Chaturangas (low planks). All of the old favourites.

This time, in the final plank practise shoulder-blade retraction and protraction to strengthen the muscles that stabilise and move them:

PLANK SHOULDER-BLADE
RETRACTION & PROTRACTION

Settle yourself into your new familiar place – a decent domed plank. Have shoulders over wrists, back long, heels stretching, hands pressing down. Once you're stable, inhale and draw the shoulder blades towards one another on your back, like you're trying to pinch a selfie-stick in between them. Exhale and separate the shoulder blades as much as you can, so they slide like tectonic plates across your back and towards your armpits.

Repeat this, ideally 10 times. Remember, nothing but your shoulder blades should move. Your chest will drop slightly as your shoulder blades draw together and rise a little as they part, but it should be subtle and should not involve the lower (lumbar) spine.

To finish, come back to a neutral place with the shoulder blades, drop the knees and take a Child's pose.

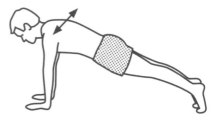

UPAVISTHA
KONASANA
Dragonfly stretch

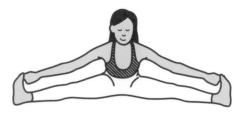

EQUIPMENT: A yoga brick
SUBSTITUTION OPTIONS: An actual brick/a cushion/a rolled-up blanket

In order to get in and out of Ashtavakrasana safely, you need to be pretty open in the inside hips. This pose – which you can do while casually reading a (i.e. this) book – will help.

Start sitting on the floor with your legs wide, a little over 90 degrees apart, with a 90-degree angle at your hip crease (if you don't happen to be carrying a protractor, that means sitting upright and not falling backwards). If you feel like you're sinking backwards, add some height under your butt (use a brick or a few cushions) until you can sit upright.

For some, sitting up with hands behind, fingers pushing into the floor, will be enough of a stretch. For others, fold forward and take the fingers to the floor in front of you, or perhaps take the hands to the shins or the feet.

As you stretch, externally rotate your legs so that the knees stay pointing upwards and don't roll inwards. Keep your glutes on, stretch through the balls and heels of the feet and don't let your sit bones leave the ground.

For some super-noodle types, your belly will come to the floor, your head will rest on the carpet and you might have a nap. If this is you, work hip stability again – make it a strength pose. Perhaps place a rolled-up towel at your hip creases so that you've not collapsed entirely onto your thighs, and rather than rest on the floor, hover your belly an inch off it and hold. Keep the butt down, resist the urge to twerk, and work your core.

Hold for 5 breaths, working up to 10. To come out, walk your hands back towards you if you're folded over, and sit up.

FIGURE 4 STRETCH

The following 3 poses are again all hip-openers, and form a slightly freakish Instagram series all on their own.

Begin with a glute and outer hips stretch. Sit with your right leg straight out in front of you on the floor, bend your left knee, externally rotate the leg and place your left foot just above (not on) your right knee. From here, bend your right leg and place the foot on the floor. You should now feel stretch in the outside of your left hip. The closer in you bring your right foot (and therefore the closer your left shin is to your chest) the more intense the stretch will be. Keeping the right foot further away from you will be less intense.

Keep your spine upright (don't collapse into a curve) – keeping hands behind you on the floor will help. Keeping your left ankle flexed will also help to protect your left knee. If you experience any pain in that left knee, back off straight away.

This stage may be enough to get into the hips for you. In which case, stay for 30 seconds, working up to a minute, breathing steadily. If this all feels good, when you're done you move to the next stage, which is Rocking the Foot-Baby.

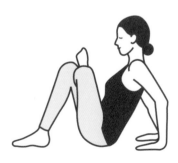

ROCKING THE FOOT-BABY & YOGA TELEPHONE

Pay attention to these pieces of fun, because they're going to make a comeback in future poses.

From the Figure 4 position loop your arms under your left thigh so that it is now resting in your elbows and draw it in towards your chest. Maybe straighten your right leg along the floor. You are now essentially holding your left leg like a baby. Rock it gently side to side. Feel the hip joy.

Stay here and breathe steadily, gently rocking, for 5 breaths, working up to 10.

The third stage is the Yoga Telephone. Once you've given your foot-child a good rock, take hold of the foot and bring it to your ear. Like you're talking on the phone. Keep your left thigh turned out from its root, and if you experience any pain in the knee or ankle, back off. Hold here for 5 steady breaths. Perhaps get someone to take a picture to prove it happened.

Repeat the whole process (starting with the Figure 4 stretch) stage by stage on the other leg, stopping at the exercise that is appropriate to both your bones and your flexibility.

BHUJAPIDASANA

Shoulder pressing pose

This is another funky arm balance that helps
prepare the hips and the wrists for Crazy 8.
Full disclosure: the final expression of this
bad boy is very much for the naturally open-hipped,
so stop at any stage of the following process. Each bit is valuable.

Start with your feet a little wider than your hips (wider still if you're broad
shouldered). Fold forward, take your hands through your legs and try to
grab anywhere along the backs of your calves (right hand to right calf, left
hand to left calf). From here use your grip to start to shuffle your shoulders
through your legs, aiming to get the backs of your shoulders eventually
behind the backs of your knees. This deeply flattering pose with your butt
in the air will help open hips and hamstrings. (Not suitable for Instagram.)

If you're fairly successfully emerging between your own legs, and can
look up at your own butt – congratulations, you've reached the next level
of yoga insanity, and you can move on to the next stage.

From this butt-gazing position, bend your knees and place your hands on
the floor behind the heels of your feet. The whole hand must be down, so
don't try to do this on the fingertips or knuckles. Bend the elbows and the
knees more if it's tricky. From here, start to take the weight in the hands
(arms are like Chaturanga/low plank with the elbows stacked over the
wrists) and make your feet light. Perhaps lift one foot off the floor. Perhaps
lift two. If both can fly, cross your ankles to lock yourself in and draw
the heels in towards you. Keep pushing the hands to the ground, keep
energetically drawing your chest through your arms.

Hold for 5 to 10 steady breaths. To come out, tip the bum down and the
feet slightly up so that you sit on the floor, then unravel your legs.

EKA HASTA
BHUJASANA
Elephant Trunk pose

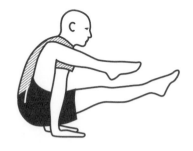

EQUIPMENT: 2 yoga bricks
SUBSTITUTION OPTIONS: 2 actual bricks,
or anything sturdy enough to take your weight

This is kind of a half Bhujapidasana, but with an element of lift and counterbalance that will help your smooth transition into full Ashtavakrasana.

Start seated with your left leg out in front of you. Take your right leg and hook the back of the knee over your right arm, as high towards your shoulder as you can. Then squeeze your arm with your leg, like a pincer.

Place your hands either side of your hips on the floor. If you have proportionally short arms, or want to make it a little easier, place yoga bricks under your hands (making sure the whole palm of the hand is on the brick).

Push down into your hands/the bricks and lift your butt up and backwards, scooping the lower belly in and doming the back. On the next breath, lift the front leg off the ground. Fly!

Try to hold for 5 to 10 steady breaths. To begin with, if it's tricky to take the leg off the floor, just hover your butt off the floor and behind you, with your front heel still on the ground. Get used to the action of pushing the ground away with the hands, doming the back and drawing in the core to lift the butt back and high.

To exit the pose, bring your beautiful butt back to the floor (gently) and remember to do the other side.

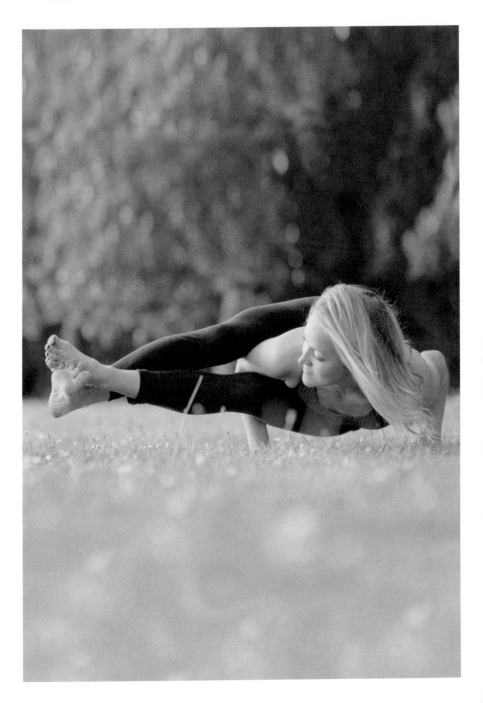

Step by Step:

HOW TO
ASHTAVAKRASANA

Once the hips are open, the arms are strong and your wrists have got used to taking your weight, it's time to go for Crazy 8 pose.

There are a few ways in and out of this pose, but for most people it's easiest to start in Elephant Trunk pose, as your leg will already be up your arm and your butt off the floor, all ready to tip into Ashtavakrasana, so it's a good idea to wait until you can levitate for a good 5 breaths in that pose before you attempt this one. When you're ready:

1. Start in Elephant Trunk pose preparation: butt on the floor, hands down by the sides (on bricks if you want), right leg squeezing onto your arm.

2. Inhale, press down with the leg on your arm, push with the arms and scoop the butt up and back.

3. Once your left (i.e. the front) foot is off the floor, bend the knee and bring it in towards you, crossing your left ankle over your right ankle.

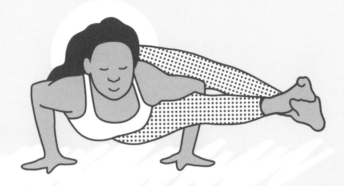

4. Once the ankles are locked in place, simultaneously tip your chest forwards, bend your arms to a Chaturanga (low plank) position and lift the butt up so it's pretty much in line with your head. Keep your right leg strongly pressing down on the top of your right arm.

5. Squeeze the inner elbows towards one another. Evert your ankles and press them together to keep them locked, and breathe.

TO EXIT: bring your butt back to earth and free your legs.

Hints & Tips

DO:

* Allow the chest to tip forwards and bend the elbows much more than you think you'll need to – it's that counterbalance that will keep your butt off the ground.

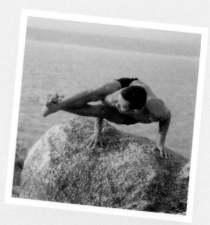

* Look up (you'll be less likely to fall down).

* Squeeze your leg like a pincer on your upper arm and squeeze your ankles strongly.

* Keep the leg as high up the arm as you can.

* Wear either fetching leggings/meggings or something long-sleeved for your arms if your limbs are sweaty. Avoid both arm and leg being bare or both arm and leg being covered. Unless you want to end in a puddle on the floor.

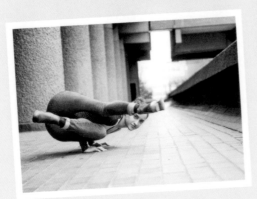

DON'T:

* Allow the elbows to wing out to the sides (if this happens then your back is not engaging and your chest will collapse).

* Drop the chest too low to the ground, or the elbow joints will be at a very acute angle, which in turn puts stress on the wrists and on the ligaments of the shoulders.

* Look up *too* high – make sure you avoid crunching in the back of your neck. If in doubt, look ahead (just not down!).

* Let the knees fall apart – engage the inner thighs.

* Sickle the hooked foot; turn the sole of the foot away from you.

TAKING IT TO THE NEXT LEVEL

Crazy 8 pose is already a fairly mental position to be hanging out in. But you can play with the angle of the legs (for example, sending the feet to the sky and letting the butt drop low), as well as trying it with straight arms (which takes more lift of the core and push of the shoulders to stop you sliding to the floor).

#Instatips

As one of the classic arm balances, Ashtavakrasana is almost always practised at height. Think gymnastic bars, railings or even just with hands holding the top handles of two heavy kettlebells. Bollards and post boxes are popular too, as are methods of transport such as bicycles and motorcycles.

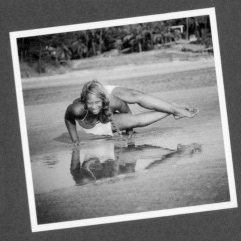

LOCATION, LOCATION, LOCATION

Urban and industrial landscapes work well with the angularity of Ashtavakrasana pose. Choosing somewhere with exposed pipework with a warehouse vibe (e.g. in east London or Brooklyn) will give you an array of background angles to play with, and usually levels and rails on which to balance precariously.

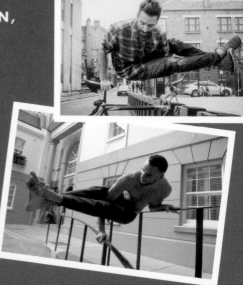

Beaches, as always, provide wonderful backdrops along with shallow waters to reflect your image back at you in the composition of your photograph.

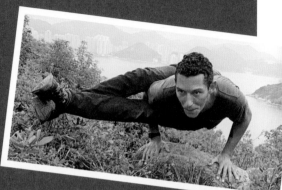

COSTUME

Loud or busy patterns will detract from the busyness of this pose, so go for something fairly plain in terms of pattern, a blank canvas on which to paint your posture. Again, dressing like a civilian in outdoor clothes will suggest a nonchalance to your impressive posing.

PROPS

As mentioned, vehicles are especially effective for arm balancing, and none more so than the bicycle. Extra community points are awarded for performing the pose on a city bicycle scheme bike, or alternatively opt for a bike with dropdown handlebars to keep with the hipster theme.

EXIT STRATEGY

If you're on the floor, simply sit the butt down. If you're balancing on a bike or on bars, this becomes more tricky. I suggest you bring a well-qualified friend to bring your butt to safety. The other alternative is to leap or handstand smoothly out of the pose (the latter can be added to your #bts Insta Story).

3/10

DANGER RATING

The SAS rating is fairly low if performed on the ground, as there is very little likelihood of any sort of falling, apart from a coccyx-smash (though in this case the Embarrassment Scale rating is high).

Performing Ashtavakrasana on a bicycle takes the SAS rating up to 7 if the bicycle is firmly chained up and leaning on something sturdy, or 8 if being held by a friend (who should be under orders to stay out of your shot). For anyone truly dedicated to the Suicidal Asana, a moving bike takes this to 10+ (though even we cannot advise this; it is the sort of stunt usually reserved for music-hall entertainment from the 1940s).

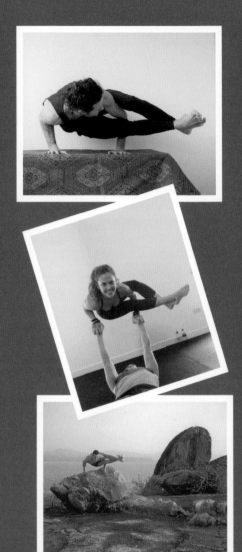

#NSFL

(NOT SAFE FOR LIFE)

Here are some yoga friends demonstrating that (a) nothing says 'holiday' like multiple poolside poses, and (b) bikinis are a must for every gender.

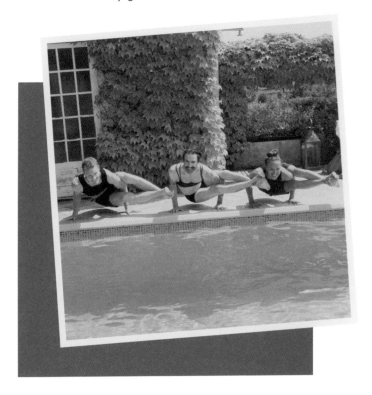

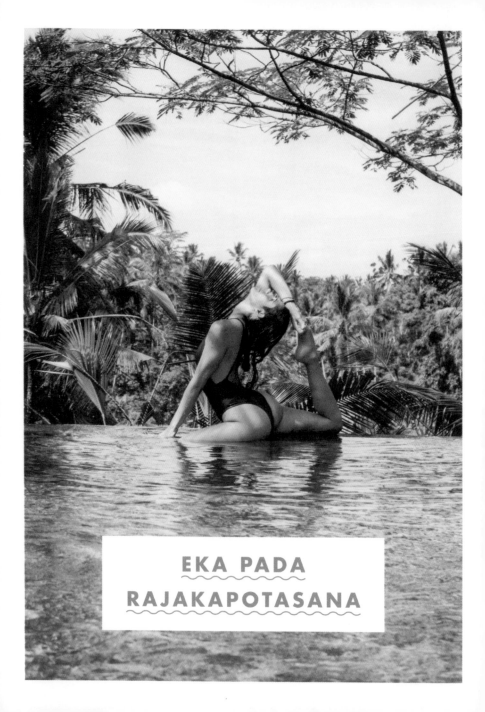

EKA PADA
RAJAKAPOTASANA

5

King Pigeon pose

Eka Pada Rajakapotasana or King Pigeon pose is one of the worst performed poses in the Insta canon. This is largely because with a little flexibility in the lower back, most people can get into some approximation of it by crunching the lumbar spine with the hips all out of whack, thus completely avoiding all the useful elements of the pose. The trouble is, unless anyone – on Instagram or otherwise (and I have yet to see an alignment-based Instagram troll) – points out there's another way of doing it, you would never know, so you keep on crunching.

When done actively, Eka Pada Rajakapotasana is considerably less (a) crunchy, (b) dramatic, and (c) pointless. If the thoracic spine is lifted and extended, there is space to breathe into the ribs, and this lift also opens the shoulders and mobilises the shoulder blades. If the core is also active, and the glutes involved, then the hips stay stable and the pelvis remains neutral rather than tipping forwards and crunching the back. Ideally, the hamstrings also contract to pull the back foot in to the body (rather than your hands manually yanking the foot in), and the quads and hip flexors stretch to allow the leg to be pulled in.

As it turns out, it's a pretty mega pose. So make sure you tune up each element with the following exercises before you put them all together.

What You Need:

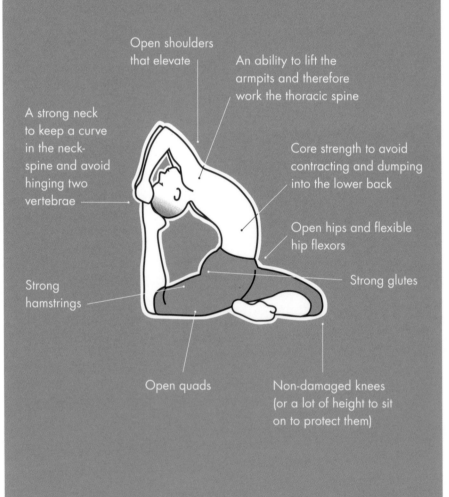

Open shoulders that elevate

An ability to lift the armpits and therefore work the thoracic spine

A strong neck to keep a curve in the neck-spine and avoid hinging two vertebrae

Core strength to avoid contracting and dumping into the lower back

Open hips and flexible hip flexors

Strong hamstrings

Strong glutes

Open quads

Non-damaged knees (or a lot of height to sit on to protect them)

Gateway Poses

ANAHATASANA

Extended Puppy pose

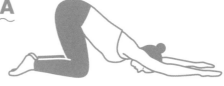

EQUIPMENT: A yoga brick or yoga blanket
SUBSTITUTION OPTIONS: Any blanket/books/cushions/folded laundry

This pose gets right into the sweet spot of the shoulders, and helps get the arms in the position you'll need for your perfect Pigeon. It is also a pose that works towards training the body to avoid a very common yoga error, of overusing lower back flexibility and underusing the thoracic (upper back) and shoulders.

For your basic Puppy pose, start in a Child's pose. Lift your hips up so that they stack over your knees and slide your chest forward and down. Don't let the hips come forwards with you. If the shoulders are tight, you may find the chest is a long way off the floor and so is the head. This is totally fine. Hang out here, with a brick or cushion under your head if you need it. If you're a little more open, perhaps the head is on the floor. For the bendy, you may also get your chest down to the floor, but be careful you're not over working your lower back – control the twerk again, so that you can open the upper back instead.

Hold this pose at whichever stage, pressing the hands lightly into the ground, lightly spinning the tops of the arm bones up and away from one another. Stay here for 10 slow breaths, working up to holding for 3 minutes.

ANAHATASANA

Extended Puppy pose with prayer (plus optional brick)

EQUIPMENT: Yoga bricks
SUBSTITUTION OPTIONS: Actual bricks/stacks of books

To work the shoulders a little more than the back, and to mimic the position of the arms and hands that Eka Pada Rajakapotasana requires, Puppy pose can be done with the hands in prayer behind the head, elbows stretching forwards away from you along the floor.

For some, resting the elbows on the floor will be enough. If it's not, place a brick under each elbow so they're raised off the floor – this will intensify the stretch.

Whichever way, try to have the skin above the elbow resting on the brick or floor, rather than the elbow point. Relax the head and stretch the elbow points away from you. Hips again stay over the knees, and the chest stretches to the floor.

Hold for 10 slow breaths, and work up to 3 minutes.

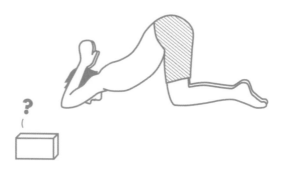

USTRASANA

Camel pose

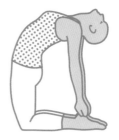

EQUIPMENT: A yoga brick
SUBSTITUTION OPTIONS: Rolled-up clothing/
cushion/pillow/cuddly toy

**Time for the legs and the gluteals. The legs are an
integral part of any backbend, so it's worth making sure they're working,
while at the same time opening the thoracic spine and chest.**

Start kneeling up. Your toes can be tucked or you can have the tops of the
feet on the floor; whichever way you feel more stable. Place a yoga brick
(or substitute) between your legs and squeeze your legs towards each
other to keep the brick held.

Next, take your hands to the gluteal creases – the crease at the bottom
of your butt cheeks where they meet the legs. This is the point you
want to move forwards in order to work the butt, stretch the hip flexors
and keep the lower back safe. So, lift your chest up to the sky ('up' not
'backwards'), and send the gluteal creases forwards. Keep squeezing the
brick between your legs and keep the core on. Feel how hard the legs
have to work to stop the back collapsing. Make sure you can still breathe.
Even Instagram Likes are not worth suffocation.

If you have the mobility (the hips are moving forwards, the hip flexors
stretching and the chest is lifting) AND the stability (you're not crunching
your lower back or cranking into your neck), take your hands down to
your heels. Keep the chest lifting. Keep the glutes on and push the feet
and legs into the ground.

Hold for 5 slow breaths. To come out, squeeze the butt, squeeze the brick
and bring the chest back upright. Sit back to your heels and rest. Work
up to taking 3 sets. A Child's pose is a nice way to end.

ANJANEYASANA

Low lunge with prayer behind back of head

This is a combination of the Anjaneyasana pose (p. 18) and the Anahatasana with hands in prayer behind the head (p. 88). This will work on the lift of the chest and opening of the shoulders as well as the required strength of the legs and the stretch of the hip flexors.

Start by setting up your Anjaneyasana. Kneel with your right foot forward (knee no further forward than the ankle) and left knee down behind you, toes of the back foot tucked under (back knee only a little over 90 degrees also). Inhale and bring the hands up over the head, stretching both sides of the waist and activating the glutes to stabilise the hips. Bring hands to prayer and drop the prayer behind you, thumbs to the back of the neck if they reach. Lift your elbows and lift your armpits and stretch the chest up to the sky (rather than back behind you, or this will again compress the back). Keep the legs active, pushing into the ground with your back foot. To make this stretch deeper and more in the shoulders and upper back, stretch the hands away from the back of the neck rather than pulling the thumbs in towards it.

Breathe and hold for 5 breaths, working up to 10. Make sure you do both sides.

To come out, squeeze the butt, push the feet down and lift the chest up in order to release. Take a Child's pose to recover.

SHIN TO THE WALL

EQUIPMENT: A yoga mat
SUBSTITUTION OPTIONS: A towel/a blanket

This is all of the juicy quad-stretch fun, preparing the front of the back leg (you might need to read that twice) for the full King Pigeon, working from the deep hip flexors to the quads.

Take a rolled-up yoga mat or a towel or blanket and find yourself a wall. Facing away from it, begin as though you're going into Anjaneyasana for what feels like the 90th time, placing your right foot forward and your left knee on the mat or towel behind you, but this time shuffle your knee right up against the wall. You're aiming to get your shin flat against the wall, toes pointing to the ceiling. Once you're in, shuffle the right foot back a little closer and sit up, taking hands to knee or hands to bricks either side of you to balance.

Have as close to a right angle in the front knee as possible, take a breath in, and on your exhale gently lift your front hip points upwards to intensify the stretch in the quads and hip flexors. Eventually you're aiming to bring the front foot back so much that you have your butt touching your heel and your back nearly on the wall, always lifting the front hip points up so you don't overly arch the back.

Try to breathe and hold for 5 slow breaths. Work up to a 30-second hold, shuffle the front foot forwards, release the back leg and rest before moving onto the other side.

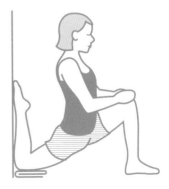

HOW TO EKA PADA RAJAKAPOTASANA

Once you've made a respectable effort to open, strengthen and lengthen, using the gateway poses, it's time to ease your way into the full King Pigeon. And I do mean ease. Go through the stages, and don't be tempted to grab at your foot and jam your head back just to touch it. This is not the object of the pose, and sadly nothing special happens when you do. Except a bit of a sore neck.

1. From a Down Dog bring your right knee to your right wrist and settle the shin bone on the floor; left ball of the foot is on the ground and the left leg is straight behind you.

2. Keep the back knee off the floor with the leg straight, and stretch your arms up overhead. This is an active 'up-Swan'. Lift the front hips up to stop crunching into the back, keep the sides of the waist long and push into the front shin. Your butt will be a good few inches (if not higher) off the ground and you should feel the stretch in the hip flexors.

3. Bend up your back leg and, using the power of your now-epic hamstrings, bring the heel of the back foot towards your butt. You now have 3 options.

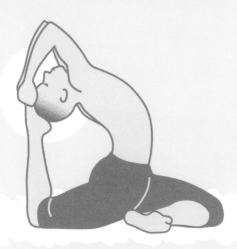

4. Option 1: Do nothing. Stay here, work the hammies, the quad stretch and the hip placement. Maybe take hands to prayer again and stretch the elbows up and the hands back. Option 2: Take a strap or belt and loop it around your left foot, lift the arms up, bend at the elbows and drop the hands down towards your back with the palms together (as though in prayer), and then walk them along the strap towards your foot. Hold on and stretch the elbows up to the sky as the foot kicks away. Option 3: Same as 2 but hold your foot in your hands.

5. Whichever option, lift the armpits and the heart and let the elbows draw back behind you rather than pulling your foot forwards (which will pull the elbows forwards as well). Push the foot up into the hands. Keep pushing the shin down and keep the glutes on.

TO EXIT: release the foot or the strap and SLOWLY bring your left foot to the floor. Rest before taking the other side.

Hints & Tips

DO:

* Place your front shin at an angle that works for your flexibility – the closer your front foot is to your hip the less intense the stretch will be; the further away it is (and the more parallel your front shin is to the front of your yoga mat), the more intense this will be.

* Keep pushing your front shin into the ground and the back foot away to the sky. Stay active.

* Look for a stretch in the shoulders, not just the hips and legs. Use a strap for as long as you need to in order to find it.

* 'Floint' your foot (point it but flex the toes) – this gives you a handle to hold or loop your strap on to and makes it less likely you'll lose the grip of your foot.

* Work towards squaring the hips, and if the hips are very wonky, consider letting your chest also follow the line of your hips, which will take any twist out of the lower back if it's uncomfortable.

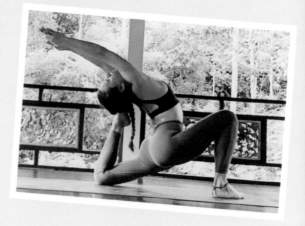

DON'T:

* Collapse the butt down to the floor and sit down unless your hips are totally square and your butt is not sticking out behind you (it is very rare that people can sit down with all of that in place). Consider sitting on a brick for a halfway place.

* Pull the back foot in so hard that the elbows come forward of the face. Actively fight with your foot; push it into your hands strongly.

* Sickle the front ankle. Actively push the grounded outer ankle down. If it's uncomfortable perhaps put a towel or blanket under it.

* Jam your head back to the foot and crunch the neck. Keep the chin parallel to the floor, looking forwards. If you must drop it back, send the chin forwards first before you drop back so you have a curve in the neck-spine and not a hinge.

TAKING IT TO THE NEXT LEVEL

If you want to up the already slightly scary broken-doll vibe . . . If you already comfortably have your foot in both hands, you can take the foot and nestle it at the back of your head, in the neck groove, leaning the head back a little to keep it wedged in, then extend your arms up to the sky with the palms in prayer (presumably praying to be let out).

#Instatips

If anything was designed for the beach, it's Eka Pada Rajakapotasana. But that said, you could perform this pose in a shed wearing a Donald Trump wig and it would still get a slew of Insta Likes.

LOCATION, LOCATION, LOCATION

Consider the shallows of a tropical pool or in the great wide sea, skin lightly peppered with sand, hair sprinkled with salt. Pools in exotic locations or shalas (yoga studios) with banana-leaf jungle backgrounds are also effective.

COSTUME

Consider a deliberate application of sand – the balance needs to be just enough to look as though you've tumbled playfully through the dunes as part of your asana, but not so much that you appear to have had a fight in it.

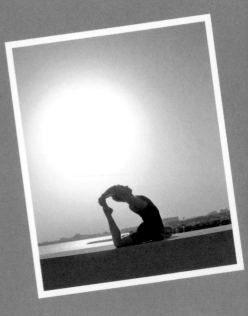

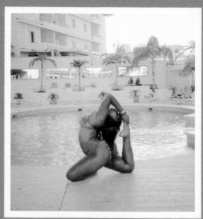

Hairography is also an important part of your picture. Consider growing hair long (for any gender), sitting in the sun, and then adding some saltwater right before the take. If your hair does not tousle and curl, you may need to set aside an hour beforehand to painstakingly wave it. Take as long as you need to ensure it looks like you took no time at all.

PROPS

Consider lining up your pose so that the sun rests upon your elbow or just above the nose of your thrown-back head. Also consider performing your pose on water rather than in it. Props such as surf boards or SUP paraphernalia make for an eye-catching floating variation.

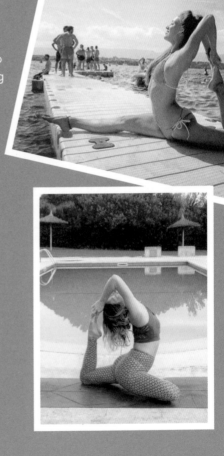

6/10

DANGER RATING

The danger of this pose stems mostly from where it is performed. All too often on beaches in Goa are people swept out to sea, taken by surprise by the element of water. Similarly, the shores of Thailand are littered with yogis having washed up off SUP boards. Perhaps ensure you have someone present to warn you of any unexpectedly large water events. Performance of this pose in surf-friendly waters (where the danger of surfboard strike is also constant) holds an 8 on the SAS.

Performance of this pose anywhere at all takes a 6 due to the likelihood of misalignment, rising to a 7 if consistently performed with wonky hips, crunched back or jammed-back head.

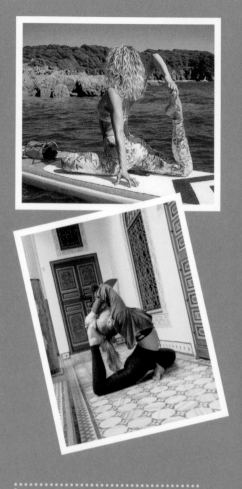

EXIT STRATEGY

If in seawater, exit during a break between the waves.

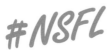

#NSFL

(NOT SAFE FOR LIFE)

Be mindful that when posing in domestic environments, objects behind you may appear to be on top of you when viewed through the camera.

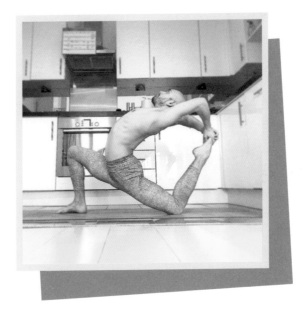

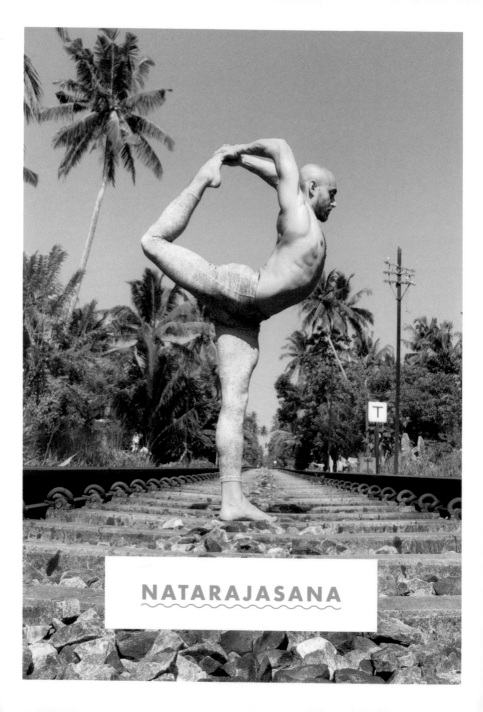

NATARAJASANA

6

Dancer pose

Natarajasana is another backbend classic. It has a number of variations, from the 'mermaid', where the foot is looped into your elbow, to the under-hand foot-grab, all the way to the double-handed over-the-top-of-the-head foot-grab.

Just like Rajakapotasana, however, it's fairly easy to get into this pose (if you have a certain degree of back flexibility) without realising that the entire body is out of line. What's most important to remember is that you really do not have to get your foot to your head, which seems to be what most practitioners are bent on doing. No one descends from on high on a magic cloud of vegan ice cream if you do.

And actually, even if you can get your foot to your head, you probably shouldn't, as you'll almost certainly be losing all of the shoulder and upper back work and throwing your hips like you're at a Shakira fan convention.

So, even if you're flexible, work on all of the gateway poses and drills. Try to get into the pose the way we're instructing here, to make sure everything that should be working is working, and everything that should be stretching is stretching – safely. If you really want to take a picture with a foot on your head, use someone else's foot. Angle it cleverly and no one will ever know.

What You Need:

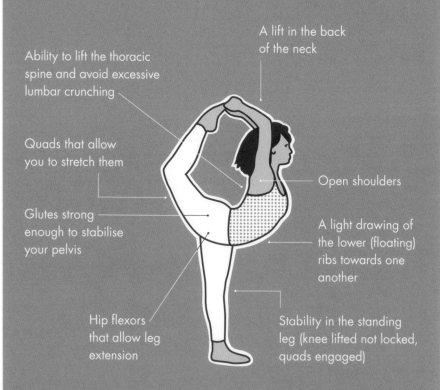

A lift in the back of the neck

Ability to lift the thoracic spine and avoid excessive lumbar crunching

Quads that allow you to stretch them

Open shoulders

Glutes strong enough to stabilise your pelvis

A light drawing of the lower (floating) ribs towards one another

Hip flexors that allow leg extension

Stability in the standing leg (knee lifted not locked, quads engaged)

Gateway Poses

As Natarajasana is a pose in the same family as Rajakapotasana (King Pigeon), all of the shoulder openers in the previous chapter will work well here. Start with one of the Anahatasana variations to get into the shoulders, and then move on to the legs with an Anjaneyasana variation.

BHUJANGASANA

Cobra pose

This pose is a good indicator of how tight your upper back may be in comparison to your over-worked lower back.

Start lying face down on the floor and take the palms of the hands to the ground, thumbs roughly in line with the lower ribs, elbows pointing to the sky.

Push the tops of your feet into the ground, and rotate the thighs internally (knees point to the floor, not out to the sides). On an inhale lift your chest, stretching it forwards as you drag your hands backwards (energetically: don't actually move them). Try to feel the work in the upper spine (not lower) and imagine the bottom tips of your shoulder blades drawing into your back. Keep the back of the neck long.

Hold for 5 to 10 breaths before slowly releasing the chest back to the ground. Take 3 rounds. If your lower back feels achy at any point, you are most likely still using the lower back muscles. Try again, only lifting the upper spine.

VIRABHADRASANA III

Warrior 3

This is a great one for strengthening the legs as well as for understanding the placement of your hips in Natarajasana.

Begin standing with the feet together. On an inhale, lift your arms over your head and lift your right knee up towards your chest, balancing on the left leg. Stay here for a breath to find your balance.

Flex the right foot at the ankle, bring your hands to a prayer position at heart centre and, as you exhale, extend the right leg back behind you and lean the chest forwards. You are aiming to look like the letter 'T', so that there is a line from your back heel to your head. Keeping your standing leg a little bent will help the balance.

As you balance, rotate your right leg (from the root of the hip) so that the big toe points to the floor and the inner thigh rolls to the sky. Squeeze your butt, especially the side glutes, and try to keep your hips in line with one another (your right hip will want to lift up).

Keeping the pelvis level, push the prayer hands together and lift the upper chest slightly, without arching the lower back. Look slightly in front of the mat with your eyes so the gaze is slightly lifted.

To intensify, release the arms and stretch them either behind you or out in front of you.

To come out, soften the supporting leg, bring the flying leg back in and to the chest, arms overhead for balance, then place both feet back on the floor.

Make sure you do both legs, and hold the pose for 5 breaths, working up to 10 breaths.

STANDING SPLITS
(closed-hip variation)

EQUIPMENT: 2 yoga bricks
SUBSTITUTION OPTIONS: Piles of copies of this book/a coffee table

This is the slightly less fun standing splits variation where, instead of whacking your leg right up to the sky, you control the angle of the hips to keep them as parallel as possible (like in Virabhadrasana III, opposite) and focus on hip stability as well as the hip flexor stretch.

Start with the feet together in a forward fold. Place your hands on the floor a foot or so in front of you, or on bricks or a low coffee table if needed, so that your legs can be straight and the hands flat. Inhale and lift the right leg to the sky. Stretch it as high as you can without allowing the right hip to lift with you. Flexing rather than pointing the foot usually helps in this variation, so you can reach the heel to the back of the room.

Keep rolling the inner right thigh up to the ceiling, so that there is a strong internal rotation of the leg and keep the butt active. Hold for 5 steady breaths, working up to 10, then release the leg back to the ground and take a little forward fold to recover before taking the other side.

DHANURASANA

Bow pose

This pose will help you access the extension of the legs from the hips as well as opening up the shoulders.

Start lying on your belly – ideally have a yoga mat or a rug/towel/soft carpet under you or this can create some funky bruises on your front hip bones. Bend your legs and bring your heels in towards your butt, squeezing the hamstrings as you do. Try not to splay the knees too wide. From here, stretch the arms and hands behind you and grab the shin bones from the outsides (thumbs facing down) right by the ankles. Ideally you should take both legs at the same time rather than one and then the other.

Inhale and push your shins back away from you – this will start to lift your chest – exhale and send your feet towards the sky. Peel the shoulders open, using the leg action. Send the chest forwards and lift the armpits up. Again, unless you're working with lower back injury or knee problems, don't let the knees escape too far away from one another. Breathe here for 5 breaths, keeping the chin neutral (don't drop the head or look too far up), pushing the pelvis into the floor, using the legs to push and the arms to resist. Work up to a 10-breath hold.

To release, relax the legs slowly, let go with the hands (without pinging out) and gently lie down. Try to do 3 sets if possible.

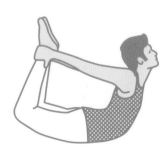

DHANURASANA
(with a strap)

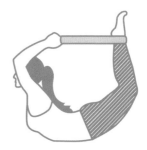

EQUIPMENT: A yoga strap
SUBSTITUTION OPTIONS:
A belt/a tie/a ribbon/a bit of rope

**This is exactly the same pose but with a different
grip of the feet, this time over the top of the head.**

Begin in the same way as the first Dhanurasana: lie on your belly with
the legs bent up so the heels are moving towards your butt. This time sit
the chest up (you can rest your left forearm on the ground for this) and,
for most, take a looped strap and with your right hand, loop it around
both feet. 'Floint' the feet (point them but flex the toes) so the strap stays
on. Lift your right arm high, bend the elbow and take hold of the strap,
keeping it looped firmly around the feet.

When you feel stable, carefully lift the left hand and also take hold of the
strap. Push the feet away and up to the sky, lift the chest and try to draw
the elbows towards one another. Just like in Rajakapotasana, do not let
your arms pull your feet in so much that the elbows are drawing forward
of your face. Push with the feet and let the arms be drawn back while
lifting the elbows and armpits up.

If you have the flexibility (in the upper back; this should not be a giant
lower back crunch), work towards smaller looped straps and eventually
no strap at all, taking hold of the feet with the hands.

Hold for 5 breaths – this can be a tricky pose to breathe through, so
make sure you don't go in too far (not breathing will be the indicator).
Try to take 3 sets with a rest in between.

Step by Step:

HOW TO NATARAJASANA

Once you've worked on the prep and feel you have a good understanding of what should be working and stretching (and what should not), you're ready for Natarajasana. It's generally a good idea to start with a strap, but you can always ditch it if it's super easy for you to reach your foot.

1. Start standing with your strap (pre-looped to a loop size that works for you) in your right hand.

2. Ground your left foot and bring your right heel up towards your butt. Loop the strap around the foot, flexing the toes of a pointed foot to keep it in place (you can reach your left hand across the body to hold the foot and keep it still as you do this if you want).

3. Once the loop is around the foot, externally rotate your right arm from the shoulder and hold the loop tightly in your hand.

4. Start to kick the foot away and up and, as you do, spin your right elbow up towards the sky until you have an over-hand grip. Then bring the left hand up to join it, holding the strap so that both elbows point upwards. Keep pushing the foot away.

5. Engage the butt, lift the chest (think Cobra), and try to even out your hips (think Virabhadrasana III). If possible, walk the hands along the strap even closer to the foot. Hold for 5 breaths.

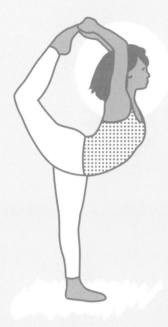

TO EXIT: walk the hands back along the strap away from the foot until you can release it safely without pinging out of the pose. Take a forward fold to release the back.

EXTRA:

To take the foot with the hands straight away (without the aid of a strap) you will need to start by reaching the left hand across the body to hold your right foot in place while you externally rotate the right arm and grab the foot with the thumb on the big toe side of the foot. Then as you push the foot away spin the elbow out and up to the sky, as you would with the strap, and bring the left hand up to join the same way.

Hints & Tips

DO:

* Keep working on lowering the hip belonging to your flying leg.

* Try to keep the chest facing forward, especially if your hips are relatively level.

* Bend the supporting leg if you need, but always keep the kneecap lifting and the muscles around it engaged.

* Flex the toes and point the foot at the same time – it will give you a ledge for the strap or a handle for your hand to hold.

* Keep narrowing the elbows – they will want to flare out wide.

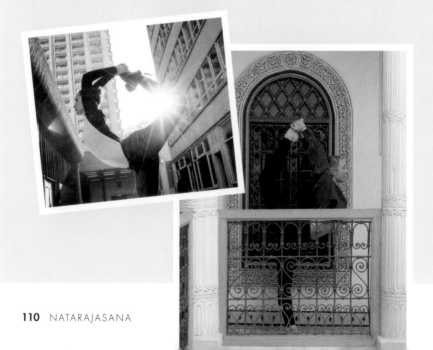

DON'T:

* Let the elbows pull forward of the face. Keep pushing the foot up and away.

* Square the chest completely if your hips are out of whack; you can allow the chest to be consistent with the direction of your hips if needs be, as this will reduce any torquing of the lower back.

* Let your chest drop too far forwards – if you're also kicking your leg high this will only intensify a crunch in the lower back.

* Lock your standing knee backward. If you do straighten it, make sure you're lifting the skin of the knee upwards.

* Stay in the pose if (a) your lower back hurts, (b) you feel pain in the shoulders, or (c) you can't breathe.

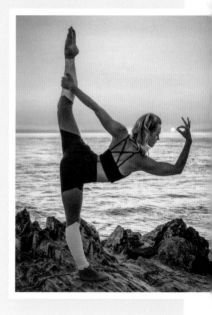

TAKING IT TO THE NEXT LEVEL

You're holding your foot in your hands near your head while standing up. There are precious few ways to take this further. Except for straightening out your back leg and holding the thigh instead. So now you're in a standing splits holding your thigh over your head. Casual.

#Instatips

This pose is wonderful in both urban and natural settings. Whether amid palm trees, waterfalls or in the middle of a busy traffic intersection in a major city, the challenge is to ensure there is enough space around you amid the throng of pedestrians, jungle trees or crashing water to let your inner stillness shine.

LOCATION, LOCATION, LOCATION

Remote waterfalls in Bali are the most popular and successful locations for standing backbends like Natarajasana. In fact, should you too make this choice, we suggest a night shoot, to make use of the moon, and to avoid the overwhelming competition for space from Instayogi crowds.

Or if you opt for daytime and an urban setting, consider lining up the sun behind your knee or in the arch of your back, somewhere

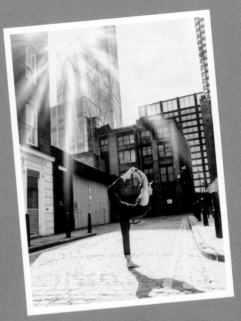

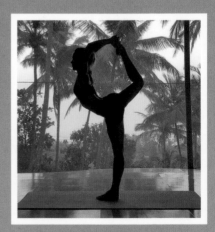

surrounded by tall, imposing architecture. For extra points/ Likes, position yourself so the sun is reflected towards the camera by a shining skyscraper behind you.

Also, never assume Instayoga is a summer game – even the ski slopes can be a photo op, especially if you keep the skis on to add an extra dimension above your head.

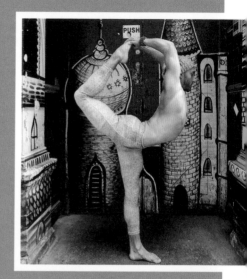

COSTUME

As with most backbends, beachwear is ideal. For waterfall shots, swimsuits, trunks and bikinis will show the line of your hips and the arch of your upper back. For men, consider pairing meggings with a baseball cap to show you have a sense of humour.

PROPS

Being thoroughly drenched (in a sexy way) or lightly glistening with water is important in the backbend genre. If you don't want to get in the actual waterfall, at least spray yourself down a little beforehand.

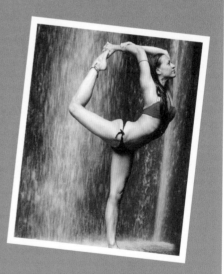

DANGER RATING

Taking hold of your limbs and keeping hold of them in water is tricky. Add in the uneven and mossy surface of waterfall rock and this pose scores an 8 out of 10. If performed in traffic, it can reach as high as a 9, assuming we're dealing with law-abiding, traffic-light-obeying citizens. In countries where stopping at traffic lights is apparently optional, this pose can reach a level 10.

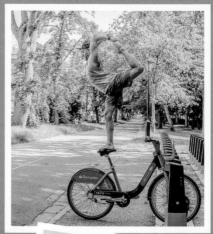

EXIT STRATEGY

When you are fully immersed in the spiritual meditation of this pose, there is a good chance you will become oblivious to the material world, which includes traffic. If you choose the urban mid-traffic setting, employ a friend to shout, 'GET OUT OF THE ROAD' when required.

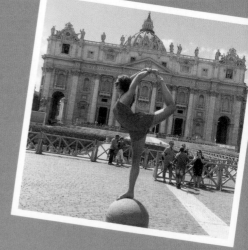

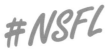

#NSFL

(NOT SAFE FOR LIFE)

Kudos for this one. Board, big shoes, small stick, big drop. We're only including this one because she's wearing so many clothes, and that transgresses the nakedness rules of Instayoga.

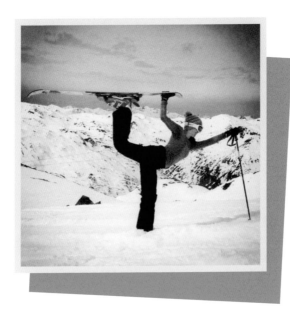

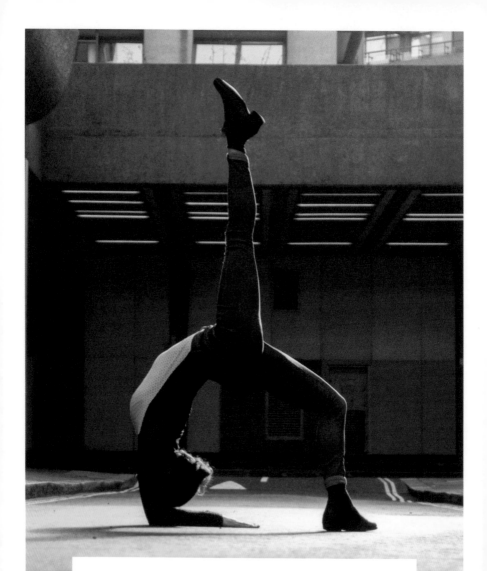

VIPARITA DANDASANA

7

Forearm Wheel pose

Viparita Dandasana or Forearm Wheel pose is a variation of full Wheel pose (or 'crab pose' as it was when you were in the playground), in which the elbows rather than the hands are on the floor. Legs can be straight or bent, and if you want to get fancy you can lift one leg to the sky. As one of the ever-popular backbends, it is another danger area for the super bendy, this time for those with a lot of mobility but not much stability in the shoulders (this combination can often lead to a stiff upper back – if one area is unstable another often holds or tightens to compensate).

The challenge for the tight-shouldered is to go slow and try to keep breathing; the challenge for the loose-shouldered is to pull back and not allow yourself to over-extend. But even if you can get into this pose and push the chest through, it doesn't necessarily mean you should. Be aware of the angle of the shoulders and be vigilant for any sensation of compression in the shoulder girdle. Follow the drills and gateway poses to strengthen as well as open the areas you need to bust out this pose safely.

What You Need:

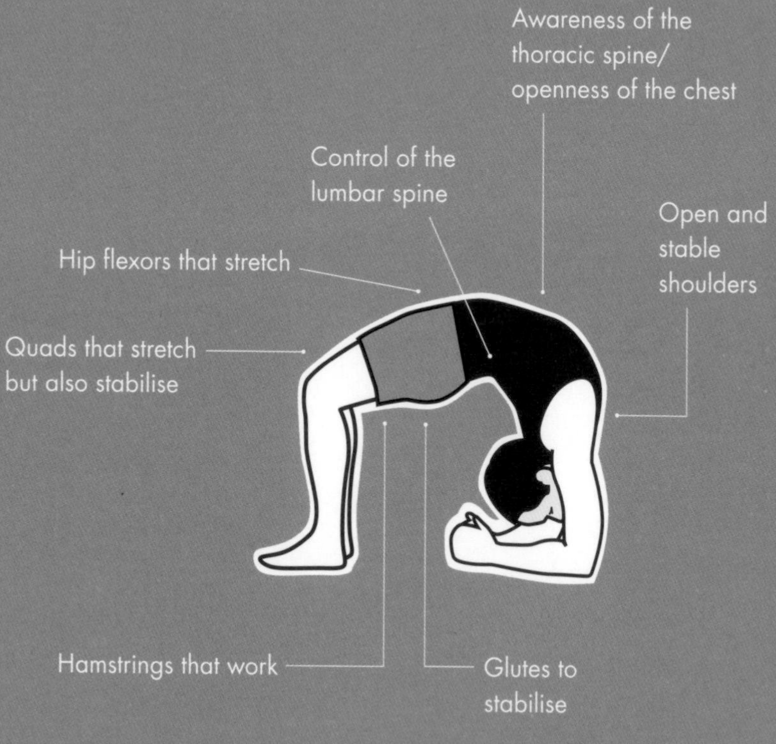

Awareness of the
thoracic spine/
openness of the chest

Control of the
lumbar spine

Open and
stable
shoulders

Hip flexors that stretch

Quads that stretch
but also stabilise

Hamstrings that work

Glutes to
stabilise

Gateway Poses

As this is yet another pose in the flattering family of backbends, all of the poses and drills in the previous two chapters will be useful, but the following are a few more to add to your armoury. This time we're paying attention to stability of the shoulders and a different position of the legs.

ANAHATASANA

(against a wall with a block)

EQUIPMENT: A wide yoga block (flatter and larger than a yoga brick)
SUBSTITUTION OPTIONS: A large hardback book/a shoe box

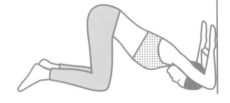

Yes it's Puppy pose. Again. With its seemingly limitless variations.

Start standing near a wall with a rectangular yoga block. Bend the elbows and hold the block between them, palms facing away from you. Walk up to the wall and place your forearms (still holding the block between the elbows) on the wall. Bend forwards from the hips (careful not to twerk the booty if you're a lumbar-jacker) and shuffle the feet back and the chest lower and lower until your chest is parallel to the ground. You will look like an upside down 'L'. →

Keep the neck long, push the forearms into the wall and squeeze the block between your elbows. Hold for 5 breaths, working up to 10, and repeat 3 times.

The next, more intense variation is to get down on the floor and repeat but this time in the Anahatasana position. So kneel down, walk your elbows to the skirting board, fingers point to the ceiling, block between the elbows again. Then shuffle the knees away and lower the chest, if possible to the ground. Hips stack over the knees (like the Anahatasana variations in the previous chapters). If that's too intense, try walking the knees further away from the wall.

Breathe (at least try) and squeeze the inner elbows towards one another, being careful not to take all this stretch in the lower back.

Hold for 5 breaths, working to 10, and try to repeat 3 times. To exit, shuffle knees further away from the wall, release the block and take a Child's pose.

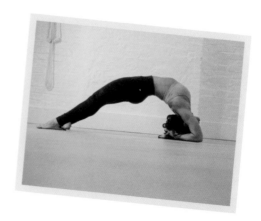

LUNGE WITH GOMUKHASANA ARMS

EQUIPMENT: A yoga strap
SUBSTITUTION OPTIONS: A belt/a tie/some string

This one will warm up the legs a little, while also preparing the shoulders.

Start in a high lunge, right foot in front, left foot behind (back heel lifted, back knee pointing forward). Inhale and lift your left arm to the sky, bend it at the elbow and reach your hand down your back between your shoulder blades.

For the tight-shouldered, take your right arm, lift it and press your hand against your left elbow (which should be pointing to the sky), stretching it slightly down and to the right.

For the full pose, drop your right arm, bend the elbow, then feed your right hand up your back in between your shoulder blades and towards your left hand. If you can grab your own hand, do, and pull the hands away from one another. If you can't reach the hand perhaps take a strap and hold it with as much length as you need, pulling on it with both hands.

Strap or no strap, keep the chest open and try not to let any tightness in the shoulders thrust your neck and chin forwards. Keep pushing the head back into the arms if needs be.

Hold for 5 breaths, repeat 3 times on one side and 3 times on the other.

To exit, release the arms and step the feet back together.

GARUDASANA

Eagle pose

EQUIPMENT: A yoga strap
SUBSTITUTION OPTIONS: A belt/a tie/a ribbon/a bit of rope

This pose is all about the shoulders again, while also giving the glutes and quads a good roasting.

Start standing. On an inhale lift your right knee and either single- or double-wrap your right leg around your left. Although it's the thighs that wrap, you can hook the right foot around the left calf to secure yourself when you're done.

Now the legs are sorted, cross your left arm over your right in front of your chest – you have 3 options for this. Option 1: Take hands to opposite shoulders (elbows are crossed). Option 2: With left elbow point sitting in the right elbow crease, take the backs of the hands together in front of you. Option 3: Wrap the arms essentially twice (like the legs) so that the palms of the hands are together.

Whichever option, bend the knees, squeeze the thighs together and sit into a squat-like position like you're sitting on a chair (careful not to stick out the butt too much). As you do, draw the elbows down and lean the chest a little forwards. Feel the stretch in the shoulders, and work the legs and butt to keep your balance.

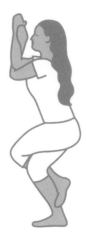

Hold for 5 breaths, and repeat 3 times each side. To exit, unravel yourself.

SETU BANDHA SARVANGASANA

Bridge pose

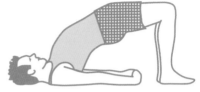

This one replicates the shape of the body (especially the legs and pelvis) of Viparita Dandasana, but with none of the tricky shoulder business to distract you from the full work of the legs and chest.

Start lying on your back, bend the knees and place your feet on the floor around hip-width apart.

Inhale and lift the pelvis off the floor by pushing into the legs, and slowly roll up through the rest of the spine one vertebra at a time. Once you get to the top, shuffle the shoulders towards one another behind you and interlace your fingers beneath your back. Stretch the knuckles away from you and push the wrists and sides of your arms into the floor to lift the chest and armpits. Activate the hamstrings by energetically (not literally) dragging the feet back towards you (feet should be stacked directly under the knees, don't move them closer) and stretching the knees away from you. The gluteal creases (that bit where your butt becomes your leg) should be lifting to the sky and the thighs energetically rolling in towards one another.

Breathe and hold for 5 steady breaths, working towards 10. Repeat 3 times. To exit, undo any binding of the hands and then slowly roll back down, trying to set each rib down individually, making sure the tailbone is the last thing to ground.

URDHVA DHANURASANA
Full Wheel pose

Full Wheel is an excellent way to work the shoulders and legs ready for Viparita Dandasana. It is also the best way to get into the pose, so it's worth making a pretty good job of it.

Begin again by lying on your back. Ideally do this following the previous exercise (Bridge pose) as one leads nicely into the other. Start the same way, legs bent, knees pointing to the sky, feet hip-width apart on the floor. This time stretch your arms up, flip the palms so they face down and place them roughly in line with your ears (your level of shoulder flexibility will determine where you place the hands, so this is just a rough guide).

Inhale, press into the feet, engage the legs and butt and lift your hips, and on an exhale push into the hands to lift the chest. If you're new to this pose, take an extra breath here with the crown of the head resting on the floor, but the legs pushing down, knees stretching away, heels drawing in. Then use your arms to lift the head off the floor and come into your full Wheel.

Work towards straightening the arms and try not to turn the fingertips in towards one another, have fingers pointed forward, or if you can, turn them slightly away from one another. Work your chest and try not to compress your lower back; imagine someone has their thumb on the back of your spine, between the shoulder blades, and is pushing upwards, so it is the chest and the armpits that stretch, rather than the lumbar.

Also, be careful of pinching the wrists – if you can't straighten your arms you may end up with a very small angle at the wrist joint – don't try to push through any discomfort if this is the case.

As for the legs, there are many variations of full Wheel pose, but for the purpose of Viparita Dandasana, try the following two.

First, the variation with heels flat to the ground. Just as in Bridge pose, have the feet not so far away that the legs straighten, but not so close that the lower back is pinching. Lengthen the lower back and again, without physically moving them, drag your heels in towards your hands and stretch the knees away. Roll the thighs internally and try not to let the knees get too wide. Use your butt – gluteal creases again should be pushed forwards and to the sky.

For the second variation, come to your tiptoes. This way the stress is taken out of the lower back and you can get a deeper stretch in the hip flexors, but the work is a little different in the legs.

Take 5 steady breaths and then bring the chin to the chest as you bend the elbows and slowly come down. Take 3 to 5 repetitions. The stronger you get, perhaps just bring the crown of the head down between sets rather than coming all the way to the floor.

When you finish, lie on your back and hug the knees to the chest, or take a gentle supine twist: for example, dropping both knees to the right with the feet wide, then both knees to the left.

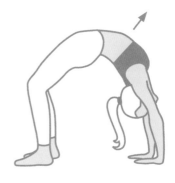

Step by Step:

HOW TO VIPARITA DANDASANA

Once you can hold a full Wheel pose (feeling the opening of the chest and shoulders) without collapse or pain in the lower back, you can move towards the forearm variation, Viparita Dandasana.

Again, this takes strength as well as openness in the shoulders, so do go slow, and if any of the gateway exercises have shown up an imbalance (e.g. that you're very mobile but not very stable), then work on the element you need to make sure you're not putting your shoulders and ligaments at risk by jumping into the full pose too soon.

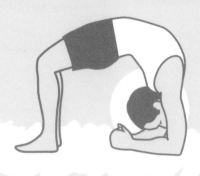

1. Start in a full Wheel. Heels down and dragging towards you. Knees stretching away from you. Lower back long.

2. Using your arm strength, slowly lower the crown of your head to the ground.

3. Once your head is resting on the floor, bring one elbow then the other to the floor. Some like to interlace the fingers behind the head, others will prefer palms flat to the ground, elbows roughly as wide as your shoulders.

4. Inhale, push into the forearms and lift the head off the floor.

5. Keep sending the chest towards the sky. You can stretch the chest through the arms a little, but if you have very open shoulders don't push this too much. Think of pulling the heads of the arm bones into the shoulder joints to avoid them rolling out of place, and push the forearms strongly into the ground. You can walk the feet away a little and straighten the legs, or you can keep them bent. Whichever way, keep the legs active. Keep the glutes on. Keep breathing.

TO EXIT: place the head back on the ground, place the hands back on the floor one at a time, push back up to a full Wheel, then bring the head down and the rest of the back and finally the pelvis to the ground.

Hints & Tips

DO:

* Find a distance for your feet that works for you – ideally have the ankles under the knees, but if you need to move the feet a little further out you can.

* Find a width for your knees that works for you – ideally knees are in line with ankles, but if the lower back is complaining, a little wider is fine; just keep the action of hugging the thighs in.

* Release the neck. Try to separate (useful) effort in the chest, shoulders and arms from (not useful) tension in the neck and jaw.

* Try to hug the elbows towards one another.

* Keep pushing down with the forearms.

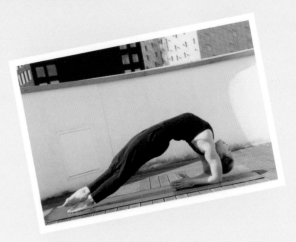

DON'T:

* Collapse and crunch into the lower back.

* Force the chest through the arms.

* Let the legs turn off and go to sleep.

* Let the elbows splay out sideways.

* Stay in the pose if the shoulders or back are pinching.

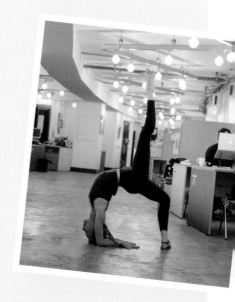

TAKING IT TO THE NEXT LEVEL

As if dropping to your elbows upside down and pressing your chest to the sky weren't enough, there are other ways to enhance your Forearm Wheel experience. You can lift a leg to the sky (go slow and make sure you keep the butt active and the supporting leg stays firm and doesn't wave out to the side); you can walk the legs away from you and straighten them out (making sure the stretch is in the upper chest and not pinching the lower back or over-extending the shoulders); and you can even lift a leg, push off the grounded foot and find yourself in a Pincha Mayurasana or Forearm Stand (which coincidentally is the next pose we'll be tackling).

#Instatips

As we know, backbends are a perennial classic in the Insta scene, so it's difficult to get this pose wrong photographically.

LOCATION, LOCATION, LOCATION

Beaches, gardens and areas of urban interest are popular. So is a moody roof. This pose can be taken with straight or bent legs, both legs down or one in the air, even holding on to the feet if you really want to show off. The single-leg variation is particularly effective amid interesting architecture, and the leg can be elevated straight to the sky or into 'over-splits' for a modern angle.

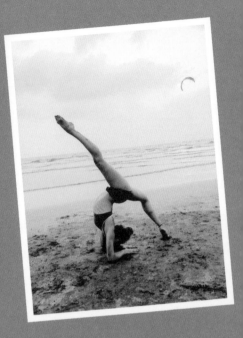

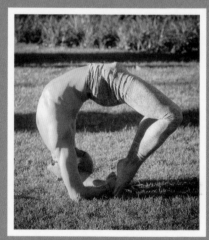

COSTUME

As usual, the fewer the clothes the better. Beachwear, bikinis, trunks, shirtless men, etc. In general, if you must wear clothes, make them tight so you can see the curve of the back and the extension of the legs. If you're wearing shoes you'll want a soft sole so that you can point your foot, or if you're in boots, ensure you can flex the foot deliberately. No one likes a half-pointed foot.

PROPS

Wrapping yourself up in fairy lights can make for a sparklingly different picture while also emphasising your lines. Plus it's a little-known fact that wearing fairy lights is very slimming.

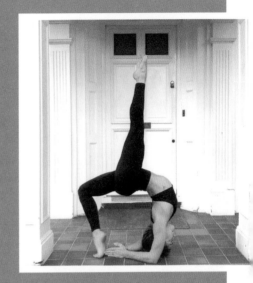

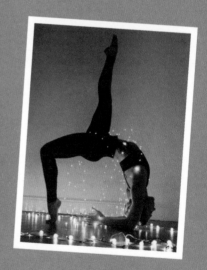

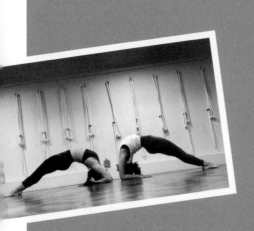

DANGER RATING

7/10

There is little danger of falling out of this one. There is danger, however, of destroying the ligaments around the shoulders, causing ongoing crippling discomfort in the lower back and straining the neck. For this reason it scores a 7.

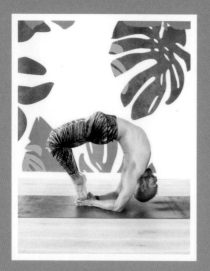

EXIT STRATEGY

Bringing the head back down to the ground is usually the best way to negotiate any sort of exit (ideally softly), and pushing back up to a full Wheel is the safest option for the shoulders. The full collapse to the floor can always be styled out as an early Savasana (or Corpse pose), the final resting position of most yoga classes, and you should stay here until any bystanders move on. This pose is also in itself an exit strategy, from Pincha Mayurasana (or Forearm Stand), which is our next chapter.

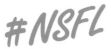

#NSFL

(NOT SAFE FOR LIFE)

If just one variation of lifting a leg or grabbing an ankle isn't enough, why not try all of the variations simultaneously?

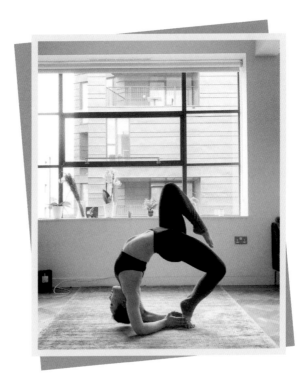

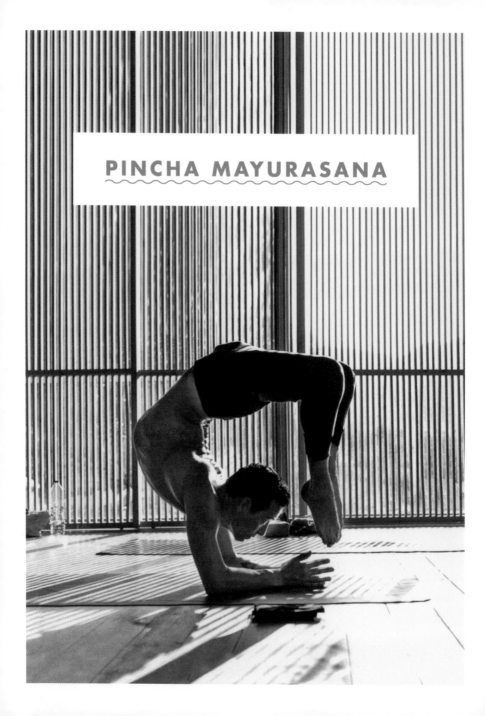

PINCHA MAYURASANA

8

Forearm Stand pose

Pincha Mayurasana is the nemesis of many, and the favourite of the few who've nailed it.

The problem with Pincha is that it involves very specific strength and flexibility. If the shoulders are strong but too tight, the face looms forward and hits the floor. If the shoulders are open but a little weak, you are likely to flip and your back will end up on the floor .

The work towards Pincha is therefore largely about balancing strength and stability of shoulders, back and core, and keeping your pelvic placement.

Once you're in, there are multiple (highly photogenic) variations of the hand, back and arm position. We will touch on a few, as the strength and flexibility of the shoulders will largely dictate which position will be best for you. Eventually you will be able to work towards being able to switch between them.

We will mainly focus on the straight-back variation rather than a scorpion-back, however, as for those bendy-backed practitioners, working continually into the backbend will not be so useful, and is usually the cause of flopping out of the pose in the wrong direction.

What You Need:

Strong legs and glutes

Long hamstrings to help smooth the ascent

Strong core to prevent over-arching the back (or falling)

Strong back

Stable shoulder blades

Open shoulders

A sense of balance

An awareness of not overusing your neck

Gateway Poses

Any of the shoulder-opening poses we've already covered (yes, Anahatasana) will be useful for this pose, and all of the shoulder-strengthening ones too, as will hamstring-lengtheners from the chapter on Hanumanasana. And here are some more to add to your armoury.

VASISTHASANA

Forearm plank

Everyone's favourite: a forearm plank. When done well, this will stabilise all the muscles around the shoulder blades and shoulder girdle, as well as strengthening the core and stabilising the hips and pelvis.

Start on your knees with your elbows to the ground, shoulder-width apart, and palms down to the floor. If possible, have your wrists in line with the elbows, fingers pointed forward, and try not to bring the hands in towards one another (unless the shoulders are so tight that you have to).

Tuck your toes, inhale, lift the knees and come to a plank. All the same cues apply as in the straight-armed plank: doming of the back, protraction (widening) of the shoulder blades, core drawing in, glutes on, tailbone lengthened and pelvis not too high or too low. Try to keep the shoulders stacked over the elbows and breathe for 5 to 10 breaths.

To exit, just lower the knees to the ground and take a Child's pose. Repeat 3 times with rests in between.

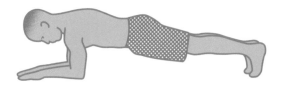

VASISTHASANA

Side forearm plank

Same pose, different view. Even more fun.

Start in the forearm plank just described, then roll onto the outside edge of your right foot and stack the left foot on top of it, keeping the right elbow on the ground and stretching the left arm to the sky. Try to keep the palm facing down to the ground and the fingers still pointing forward, only allowing the hand to draw into the centre line a little if you really have to for the shoulder. The aim of keeping the fingers pointed ahead is to key into serratus muscles and externally rotate the shoulder; letting the hand wander in often internally rotates the shoulder instead.

Breathe in your side plank. Imagine trying to wrap your right shoulder blade underneath your right armpit. Keep the legs strong and lift the left hip towards the sky. Either keep the left arm stretching up or stretch it towards the front of your mat to help you lift the hips, like a sideways banana.

Try to hold for 5 breaths, working up to 10. Don't let the hips collapse down or the top hip roll backwards and open. Keep the hips stacked one on top of the other. If the left hip tends to fall back (making your pelvis roll to face the sky), you can always step your left foot in front of your right instead of having one stacked on top of the other. This will prevent the hip roll.

To come out, slowly drop the left arm to the floor coming back to forearm plank, drop the knees and rest. Repeat 3 times.

DOLPHIN POSE

(3 hand positions)

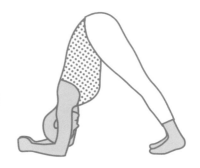

Dolphin pose is an excellent way to build strength, open the shoulders, and find the position you will need to be in or near for your full Forearm Stand.

Start on your knees with your elbows on the floor. There are 3 hand positions to try: each one requires recruiting slightly different muscles, but more importantly, they require different levels and angles of shoulder flexibility.

We'll start with the position most people find the most accessible, which is with the hands together, fingers interlaced so that the sides of the forearms and the little finger side of the hands are on the floor. With all of these, do not let your elbows creep out wide. Just like in the forearm plank, think of hugging your elbows in towards one another.

Now, pressing firmly into the arms, inhale and lift the knees. Work towards straight legs, but how straight they get will depend on your hamstring flexibility (so keep them as bent as you need). Keep on the balls of the feet and tiptoe the feet as close in as you can, working towards stacking your hips over your elbows. As you do this, notice how your shoulders will probably want to drop forwards along with the chest. Resist by pressing the chest back towards the legs and trying to keep your shoulders over your elbows, not forward towards your hands. Breathe here for 5 to 10 breaths, then drop to the knees and rest. →

The second hand position is again with the elbows about as wide as the shoulders, with palms this time flat on the floor, but bring your thumbs to touch, so that the arms make a triangle shape on the floor. Then repeat the remaining steps described for the first position.

The third hand position is usually the most difficult for those with tight shoulders, especially those press-up kings and queens who have very developed pectorals but perhaps not such a strong back. For this one, just like for the forearm plank, elbows are as wide as the shoulders, palms are on the floor, but hands are in line with the elbows, like train tracks. Again, repeat the remaining steps.

Relax the head in all of them, looking through to the feet if you can, to make sure there is no tension or gripping in the neck. Don't let the elbows stray apart like Bambi, and don't let your face hit your hands – keep pushing the chest back towards your legs and pushing the floor away with your arms.

Hold each version for 5 to 10 breaths, doing each exercise once or perhaps just one of them 3 times.

MOVING DOLPHIN

Who knew Dolphin pose could get even more enjoyable?

Adopt Dolphin variation 1 or 2, so the hands are in some way together, with a triangle shape of the arms. Once you're in, on an inhale look towards your hands and bring your nose towards your thumbs (i.e. all of the forward moving of shoulders and chest that you DON'T want to be doing in your Dolphin pose), and on the exhale send your chest back towards the legs as far as you can. Repeat: inhale to bring the shoulders forward and nose towards your thumbs, exhale to push the ground away and send the chest back towards the legs.

Repeat this, working up to 10 times forwards and back. Focus more on the back element – taking the chest towards the legs – rather than trying to get too close to the floor in front of you. The important element is the strength to take the chest away from the ground; the coming forwards is just giving you the opportunity to do that.

To exit, as with Dolphin drop the knees and sit back to the heels. Rest. Work up to doing 3 sets of 10 back and forths.

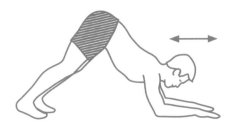

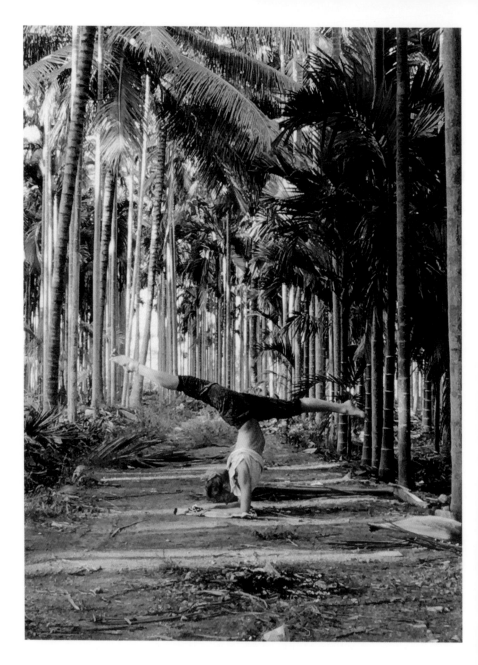

ANAHATASANA

(against wall with strap)

EQUIPMENT: A yoga belt
SUBSTITUTION OPTIONS: A belt/a scarf/a bit of old rope

YES! It's another Anahatasana. This one is again using the wall, but the action is a little different.

To begin with, practise this standing up. Take a strap (or scarf or belt, etc.) and head to a wall. Put your forearms on the wall, elbows shoulder-width apart, hands in line with elbows, fingers pointing up to the ceiling. Hold the strap between thumb and index finger on each hand. Pull apart, like you're trying to move your hands away from each other (but they won't move, because you're tightly holding the strap). Try to start this action from the back – from the bottom of the armpits and shoulder blades – rather than thinking about it being an action of the hands or arms.

To do the full pose, face the wall, drop to the knees and adopt your best Anahatasana. Ideally hips stack over the knees, but you can move the knees as far back as you need. Take your elbows to the floor and shuffle them right up to the wall. Forearms are against the wall, fingers pointing to the ceiling, elbows shoulder-width apart and hands in line with elbows. Stretch the chest down to the floor. Now repeat the action: take the strap in the hands and try to rip it in half, pulling the hands away from each other. Work from the armpits and shoulder blades.

Breathe and hold for 5 breaths. Rest by releasing the strap, sinking the butt to the heels and taking a Child's pose. Work up to taking 3 rounds.

Step by Step:

HOW TO PINCHA
MAYURASANA

Once you can perform the gateway poses
without shaking, quivering and needing to
take a day off to recover, you're ready to
try working towards Pincha Mayurasana.
Remember though, this pose requires so
many very specific elements of both strength
and flexibility that for most people it will be
a fairly long time coming. Of all the poses,
in fact, this one takes most people the
longest to master.

When you start practising Pincha
Mayurasana, it is a very good idea to
do this against a wall. Coming out of
Pincha is an art form in itself – trickier,
even, than cartwheeling out of a
handstand, for instance. So use a
spotter or a wall until you're confident
you can come up and down with
control and save yourself.

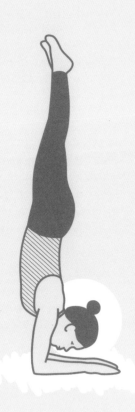

1. Find a wall if necessary. Drop to your knees and place forearms on the floor, adopting any of the Dolphin hand positions on pp. 139–40 ('traditional' Ashtanga Pincha has the hands in line with the elbows, but while you're learning, start with the one that gave you the most stable and accessible Dolphin pose).

2. Tuck the toes, lift the knees and walk the feet in as close as you can to your elbows.

3. Lift your favourite leg to the sky as high as you can. Point it to the ceiling and engage your butt.

4. Soften your standing leg, inhale and take SMALL hops off the leg, using the flying leg as your guide (specifically the butt of the flying leg – keep it squeezing). Point the leading leg where you want to go, push the ground away with the hands, and keep the core on.

5. To begin with, you are just looking to delay the landing of your hopping leg for longer and longer, but once you find a balance, keep the legs split still – that way you have control to tip more or less forwards or backwards. Only bring the legs together in the air when you feel fully balanced, and when you do, control your pelvis, bringing the hips towards your ribs.

TO EXIT: split the legs again and bring one foot at a time back to the ground.

Hints & Tips

DO:

∗ Control your elbows: don't let them splay outwards or your face will get closer and closer to the floor. Which is not ideal in this scenario.

∗ Avoid jutting your chin forward and craning your neck. Looking back to your feet will feel scary at first, as you can't see where you're hopping to, but even if you don't want to look back, modify the looking forward, and be aware if you're pulling into your neck.

∗ Step your feet as close to the elbows as you can before you start hopping, and keep the top leg super active.

∗ Think of the back of the sacrum lifting up rather than just the leg – this should stop you over-arching the back.

∗ Squeeze both legs together if you come up – your legs support your spine even when you're upside down.

∗ Make sure you do both legs. Even the rubbish one.

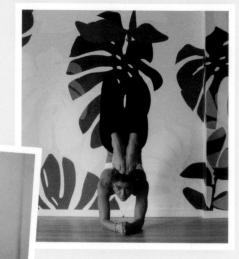

DON'T:

✳ Get impatient after a few controlled hops and suddenly fling yourself into the air. Momentum will get you nowhere but flat on your back, or fixing a new hole in your wall.

✳ Stick your butt out in order to find counterbalance. Bring the front hips lightly towards the ribs.

✳ Stick the ribs out – lightly draw the lower ribs towards your front hips, making sure you can still breathe.

✳ Point your hopping foot too fiercely – if it's not lifting that high off the ground, it will pull you back down. Focus on the flying leg.

✳ Bring the legs together too soon – keep the splits and work on the balance.

TAKING IT TO THE NEXT LEVEL

For poses like Pincha there are myriad variations. Scorpion Pincha involves bending the knees and bringing your feet towards your head while arching the back, lifting the head and bringing the chest parallel to the ground, until eventually your feet are resting on your Insta-friendly hairdo.

You can also take leg variations – once you're up you can wrap the legs around one another in Eagle pose; or you can take the legs into Lotus pose (Padmasana) and keep the knees to the sky, or, if you're feeling brave, you can lower the knees down towards your armpits. Ashtanga practitioners (those who practise the strict Vinyasa form of Ashtanga Vinyasa) get very excited about this.

#Instatips

There are so many opportunities for Instagram glory with this pose once you have the control. The legs can be together, apart, at funky angles or wrapped in Lotus position. Then there's the back position – you can take it to Scorpion, to a hollow back, or find your arrow-straight line. The Insta-pose world really is your open-shouldered oyster.

LOCATION, LOCATION, LOCATION

Poolside 'candid' pictures, as though someone just caught you in the middle of an intensely meditative flow, make for great and highly enviable Instapics. Make sure the full extent of the luxuriousness of your location is clear from the picture (infinity pools, astonishing views, cloudless azure skies, etc.). Beaches and tropical backgrounds are, of course, always a win, as are

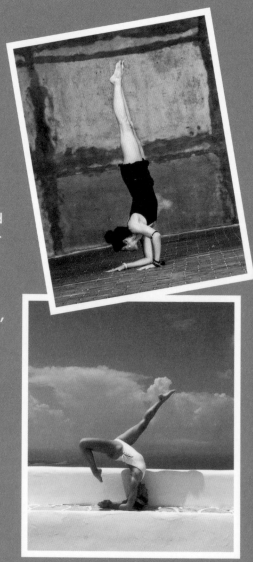

urban warehouses and textured or coloured backgrounds like slatted wood or green walls.

COSTUME

For the Scorpion variation, with the feet dangling over your nose, consider unlikely footwear, like a wedge heel. Combining this with a deliberate alignment of the sun, as mentioned in many of the backbends (perhaps at the tips of your wedge toes), can be startlingly effective.

As always, for beach and tropical shots wear as few clothes as possible. Show off your lines and consider going #shirtless.

PROPS

Consider tattoos. The majority of yogis use these as a major point of interest of their asana nowadays, so make sure you have one, or get one, or draw one on (the abdomen is a particularly good location). Above all, ensure that you shoot your picture from an angle that shows it off best.

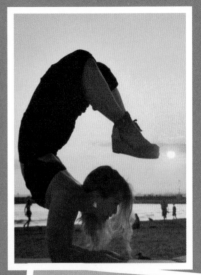

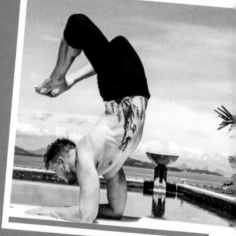

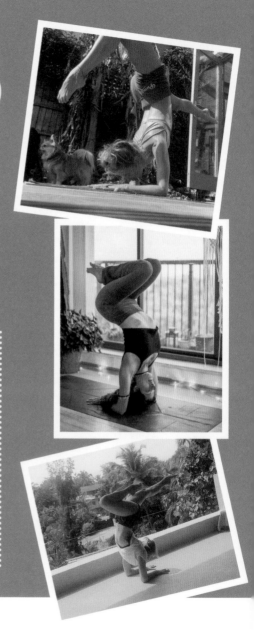

8/10

DANGER RATING

The likelihood of tumbling out of a Pincha is fairly high, but performing it on soft ground takes the rating down to about a 5. If at height, on uneven ground or attempting with interesting footwear, the rating increases to 8.

EXIT STRATEGY

If this is a poolside shot, an emergency exit into water is an excellent strategy. Beaches are soft and therefore shouldn't leave you too winded. For a more graceful exit, however, learn how to step out into Viparita Dandasana (the previous pose you nailed) like it's the easy and natural way out.

#NSFL

(NOT SAFE FOR LIFE)

There is a term in yoga philosophy, 'Pratyahara', which loosely translates as the withdrawal of the senses. When taking pictures of inversions, try to avoid the literal Pratyahara that comes from ending up with your costume over your head.

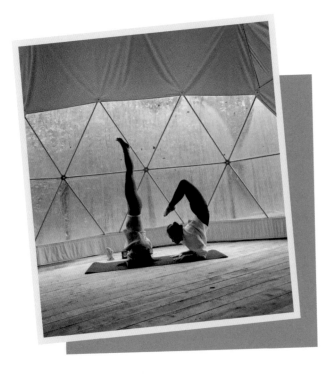

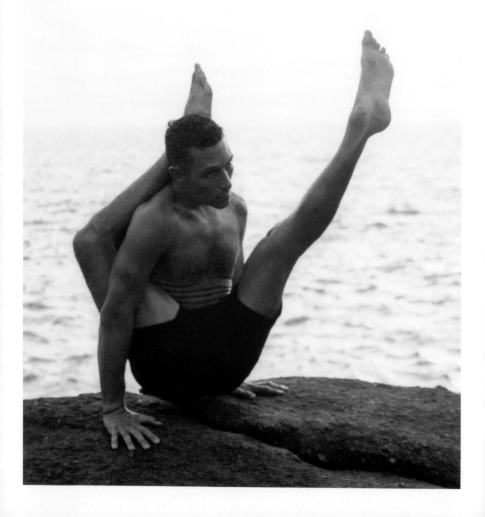

EKA PADA SIRSASANA

9

Leg-behind-the-head pose

Do you remember when you were thought of as really flexible if you could touch your toes? Well, forget that. Nowadays the basic benchmark is popping your leg behind your head.

Just to be clear before we begin, the majority of your 'skill' in this pose comes down to your natural range of motion around the hip. You can increase your flexibility to a certain extent, but ultimately, if your bones are not made for this pose, you ain't getting in.

Also, once again, just because you can do this pose, doesn't necessarily mean that you should. And certainly not regularly. If you're very mobile around your hip joint or have very little (protective) tight soft tissue, you're likely to be working into a place where bones are meeting other bones, possibly compressing bone on bone.

Ideally, this pose should be an active not a passive one – i.e. you should be able to pop that leg behind your head without having to pull it there with your hands. Just bear that in mind when you're yanking your leg up towards your shoulder . . .

What You Need:

Strength to lift the chest and draw the shoulders backwards while your foot is dragging them forwards

A good notch at the back of your neck

Stretchy hamstrings

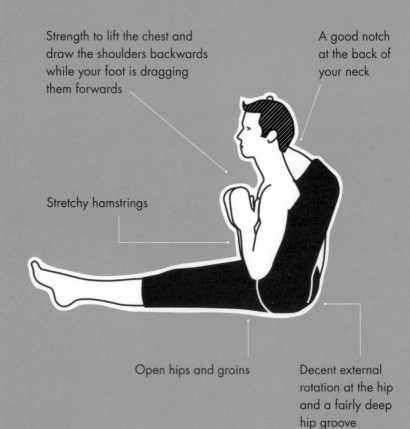

Open hips and groins

Decent external rotation at the hip and a fairly deep hip groove

Gateway Poses

So. Even if these gateway poses never get you to the full wonder of Eka Pada Sirsasana, they should both strengthen and free up your hips. As usual, listen to your screaming groin, and never push yourself to an unacceptable level of pain.

As a heads-up, Rocking the Foot-Baby and the Yoga Telephone are both important ways into the full version of this pose, so as well as the following, keep up your rocking and phoning, yogically.

BADDHA KONASANA

Active Butterfly pose

EQUIPMENT: A yoga blanket or a yoga brick
SUBSTITUTION OPTIONS: Cushions/folded sheets/an encyclopaedia (year irrelevant)

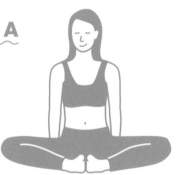

This one is a great pose for getting into the groins, while also trying to activate the glutes to make it an active rather than a passive stretch.

Sit on the floor and place the soles of the feet together with the knees wide, like a diamond shape. If you feel like you're falling backwards or you're having to strain at the hips not to round the lower back, then sit on something – a yoga brick or a couple of cushions are good. →

Place the fingertips behind you on the floor (or on something if you need more height). Push them down in order to lift the chest and stretch the back. Push the soles of the feet towards each other. Try to engage your butt while imagining sending the knees away from one another rather than forcing them down to the ground. The more you engage the glutes, the more your knee-pits should open. To understand what that sentence even means, take a thumb and place it in the space behind one of your knees (the knee-pit). Squeeze on your thumb with your leg and start to draw your thumb back out of the pit and towards the quads, allowing the skin to move with the thumb. It will look like the skin from behind the knee is moving outward, making space at the back of the knee.

If your knees are touching the floor (without forcing them there), you can take your hands to your feet and fold forward, keeping the sit bones on the ground.

Hold for 5 breaths, keeping the glutes on and the chest long. Repeat 3 times.

SUPTA PADANGUSTHASANA B
Reclining hand-to-big-toe pose B

EQUIPMENT: A yoga brick and a strap
SUBSTITUTION OPTIONS: A firm cushion/a pile of books and a tie/a belt

This pose again works into the inner hip while stabilising the hip joints. If you're already very flexible, don't be tempted to whack the leg out to the side. The important thing is keeping the hips as level as you can, not jamming the leg to the floor.

Lie on your back, take your brick or cushion and place it next to your right hip, close enough that it's touching. Inhale and bring your right leg up to the sky with your belt looped around the soft part of your foot, towards the heel. Push into the belt with your foot and pull on the belt with your hands.

Keep your leg at 12 o'clock, straight to the sky (even if you can pull it further in towards you), and push your leg away at the same time as pulling it in with the hands on the strap. Find the right balance of push and pull to keep it pointing straight upwards. Keep your butt on the floor, and try to ground the back of your left thigh on the floor.

Now it's time to get into the hip. Keeping your hip points as even as you can (you will want to rock to the right), take the ends of the strap in your right hand and open the leg out to the right. If you are very mobile in the hip, you will probably hit the brick or cushion: that is exactly what it is there for. Don't let the left butt cheek become light or the left thigh leave the floor. Keep pushing with the foot and pulling on the strap. Feel the opening in the inner right hip, but keep the leg active.

Hold for 30 seconds, breathing steadily, then bring the foot back to the centre, release the strap and hug both knees into the chest. Repeat on the other side.

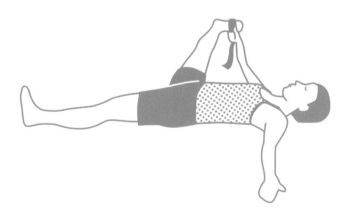

HALF HAPPY BABY POSE

EQUIPMENT: A yoga strap
SUBSTITUTION OPTIONS: A tie/a rope/ribbon/a belt

This is a direct follow-on from the previous exercise.

Repeat exactly as previously described, but once the right leg is out to the side, bend the knee and draw the knee towards your armpit, sole of the foot facing the sky. Take hold of the outside edge of your foot (little-toe side) with your right hand. The top of your right thigh will probably be resting on the brick or cushion, again this is totally fine.

Now, externally rotate the right hip (think of spinning the thigh open from the root) and resist your own hand: push the right foot to the ceiling (sole of the foot still pointing straight up) as you pull down with the hand. After 10 seconds of this, let your hand win the fight, and allow your knee to drop a little closer towards the armpit.

Hold for 30 seconds. To release, let go of the foot and hug both knees to the chest before taking the other side.

Never push through any pain in the hip joint in this one, and if holding the sole of the foot with your hand is too much, take the strap again, loop it around the foot and hold the strap with the right hand instead.

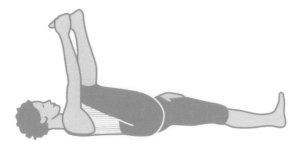

ANANDA BALASANA

Full Happy Baby pose

EQUIPMENT: A yoga belt
SUBSTITUTION OPTIONS:
A tie/a rope/ribbon/a belt

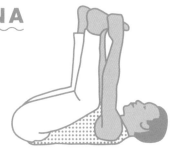

**Surprisingly enough, this works along
much the same lines as the half Happy Baby,
but with both feet at the same time.**

Lie on your back and draw the knees up towards the chest.
Perhaps spend a moment circling the knees away from one another and
then in towards one another, making small circles just to mobilise the hips.

When you're ready, take both hands to the outsides of the feet (again,
little-toe side) and draw the knees towards the armpits, keeping the soles
of the feet facing the sky and, if possible, the whole of your sacrum and
tailbone on the floor. If it's tricky to take the feet, or if the tailbone flips
up, lay a strap across the feet (dangling one end off the outside edge
of each foot) and then take the hands to the strap ends instead of to the
feet themselves.

Repeat the same pattern as for half Happy Baby: push the feet into the
hands/strap and pull down with the hands/strap for 10 seconds, then
gradually let the hands win and draw the knees in towards the armpits.

Try to keep the back long (don't curl the front hips towards the ribs,
lengthen them away from the ribs instead), keep the entire back down,
and again, don't push through any pinching or pain.

Hold for 30 seconds and then release. Hug the knees in to relax the
hips for a few breaths. Repeat 3 times.

SUPTA EKA PADA SIRSASANA

This is your full Eka Pada Sirsasana, but lying on your back, which is usually a slightly more accessible version when you first try it.

Start by lying on your back and come to a half Happy Baby pose, right leg up, left leg straight along the ground. From here, move into the Rocking the Foot-Baby exercise (p. 72): knee into your right elbow crease, holding the outer right foot with your left hand, possibly even taking the right foot into the left elbow crease.

Rock the foot and leg gently right and left, making sure you're opening from your hip joint (and putting no pressure on the knee). If this is difficult, bend up your left leg, left foot on the ground and left knee pointing to the sky.

From here move into the Yoga Telephone (p. 72), externally rotating from the right hip joint, drawing the right knee towards the floor behind you, and taking the right foot towards either your forehead or, ideally, your right ear.

Now, in an ideal world, this would be an active stretch and you would be able to get your foot to your ear without using any persuasive pushing or pulling from your hands at all. In all likelihood, however, you will need some arm-strength persuasion. Just make sure you are not yanking the leg past a safe position for you.

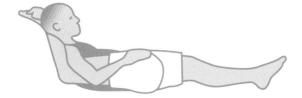

If your Yoga Telephone is progressing fairly easily, firstly, if your left leg is bent, straighten it out. Then, if this is still 'comfortable' (relative term), bring your heel towards your forehead, duck your head, and see if you can pop the head under the ankle. The back of your neck will provide a perfect shelf for your ankle to rest in. You can keep holding the right foot with the left hand if you need to, and you can send your head back into the ankle to keep it in place and to stop your head jutting forward.

If you've got yourself in, swim your shoulders through, backpacking the right leg as much as you can. With your free hand you can grab your right butt cheek. Supposedly this helps keep your right shoulder through the leg. But it's also just fun.

Hold for 30 seconds. Try to release slowly, by removing your ankle using your left hand. Lie on your back and recover before repeating on the other side.

Step by Step:

HOW TO EKA PADA
SIRSASANA

Obviously if you can't get your leg around your head when you're lying on your back, you're not going to get it around your head when you're sitting up. So with this pose more than any other, only try this if you really have found your way fairly comfortably through all of the gateway stages and postures.

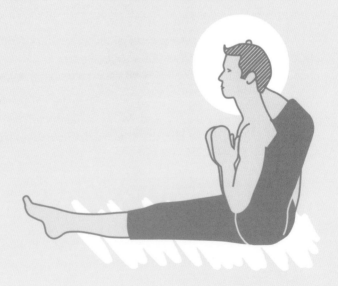

1. Sitting down with your legs outstretched in front of you, bend up your right leg and take it in your arms.

2. Depending on how warmed up you already are, you may want to take Rocking the Foot-Baby and the Yoga Telephone. Otherwise, if you have worked through all of the warm-ups and preparation, take your right leg and backpack it as high up your right arm as you can.

3. Push your right shoulder back lightly into your thigh, and roll the outer right hip towards the floor to externally rotate at the hip joint. Lift your right foot up – either towards your face or above your head using your left hand.

4. Keeping hold of your ankle with your hand, duck the head under the foot and place the ankle at the nook behind the back of your head. Draw the head back a little to prevent your head from jutting forward.

5. Try to sit up as tall as you can and, if you can let go of your foot without it pinging back out, take the hands to prayer in front of the heart, and push the elbows and upper arms back.

TO EXIT: remove your ankle using your left hand. Relax.

The other way into this pose is to take Supta Eka Pada Sirsasana, and then from your back, swing your straight (free) leg towards your face and then away from you in order to bring yourself up to sitting.

Hints & Tips

DO:

✳ Try to sit up a little once you're in, especially through the upper spine/chest – this will help lessen the weight of the leg pushing on the neck (which otherwise is taking all of the strain).

✳ Keep holding your ankle or foot behind your head with your opposite hand until you're able to get the lift of the chest (which may take some time).

✳ Push the base of the neck and shoulders back into the ankle when you do start working on releasing your grip on the ankle.

✳ Keep externally rotating from the hip joint (not the knee joint!) throughout.

✳ Bear in mind that for some people the shape of your bones and the angle of your joints might not ever let you in. This is fine. Be willing to let it go and stick with your Yoga Telephone. Which is a good enough party trick for this lifetime anyway.

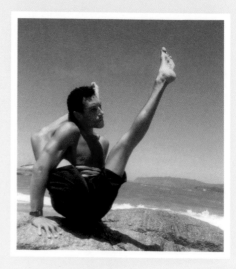

DON'T:

* Do this without a decent warm-up.

* Push through any pain or discomfort in your knee.

* Persist if it is causing pain in your neck.

* Allow your neck and chin to jut forward (again, hold the ankle as long as you need).

* Take the foot behind the head at all if you have to fight. Keep at the exercises until it becomes a movement that is within your (ideally active) range of motion.

* Ping out of the pose when you're finished – come out slowly, removing your foot manually with your hands, and try not to whack yourself on the back of the head with your foot as you do.

TAKING IT TO THE NEXT LEVEL

As well as Supta (the lying-down version) and then the seated version, from seated if your hands are free you can place them on the floor and lift your butt up. One leg stays behind your head and the other one (that was on the floor in front of you) points up to the sky – flying Eka Pada Sirsasana!

#Instatips

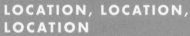

Both Eka Pada Sirsasana and the Supta (lying down on your back) variation make for pictures that will convince the world you are an advanced yogi. Have fun with these – the fact that your leg is behind your head will make up for any lack of imaginative background.

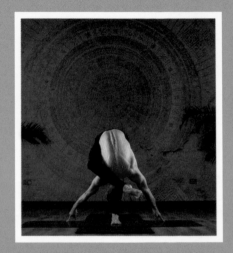

LOCATION, LOCATION, LOCATION

Photographically speaking, Eka Pada Sirsasana is in a similar category to arm balances. Once again, this pose looks particularly good at height, such as on a rock or an outcrop, but also somewhere with intense circular artwork in the background.

Alternatively, choose a background that is super simple, but flip the pose upside down and make it look super complicated.

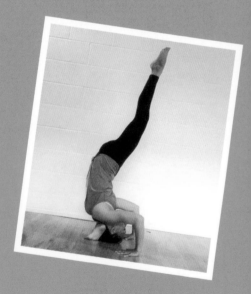

COSTUME

The costume implications for this pose revolve largely around the fabric's ability to stretch enough to get your leg where it needs to be. Also, in an exception to the 'fewer clothes the better' Insta rule, no one likes a crotch shot. Choose leggings or trousers.

PROPS

Animals are a win-win situation in an Instapic. If they behave they will break the internet with their adorableness; if they misbehave, it makes for the best blooper shot you'll get all year. Dogs are particularly popular, especially if said dog is either interfering with your practice or showing total disinterest in your epic yoga achievements.

Also consider partner yoga. Not *actual* partner yoga, which requires special skill, but the sort of partner yoga where you rope someone in (someone who's better at yoga than your actual partner) so the two of you can perform a

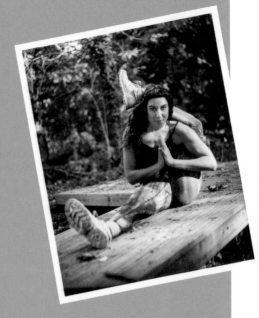

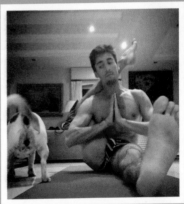

pose in tandem. You can sit side by side, laugh at one another's perfect posture, and look into one another's slightly strained eyes. This sort of partner yoga shows the world you're super fun and hilarious, even when doing yoga.

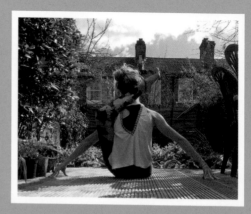

DANGER RATING

The danger in this pose largely stems from the likelihood of thwacking yourself in the face with your own foot. For those with elastic hips, this pose scores a 6 on the SAS purely because of the tricky exit. And although this pose has a fairly low imminent-death rating, the chances of messing up knees, necks and hip joints are fairly high if the pose is done often and without due care and attention. In the long term, this pose scores a 7.

7/10

EXIT STRATEGY
Carefully.

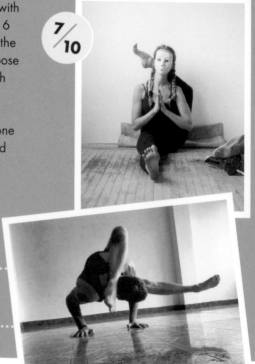

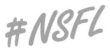

#NSFL

(NOT SAFE FOR LIFE)

Although Instayoga is an excellent chance to show off your mastery of both yoga and life (and hair and outfit choice), you can also thrust others into the limelight, by achieving a pose on their behalf.

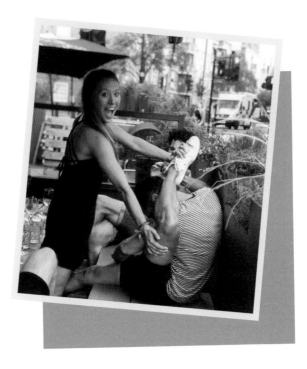

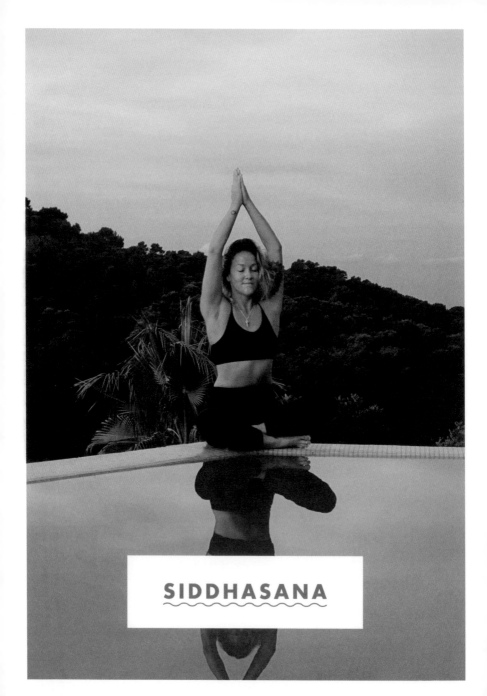

SIDDHASANA

10

Perfect pose*

After all of that hip opening and back bending, it's time to do some serious sitting. Siddhasana, also known as 'accomplished' or 'perfect' pose is considered one of four important meditative positions. It's second only to Padmasana, Lotus pose, but has the benefit of allowing most tight-hipped people to get somewhere close to approximating it without ruining their knees.

Don't be fooled, though, by the apparent ease of this pose. Sitting for long periods, or even relatively short ones, can be surprisingly painful, as anyone who has flown on a budget airline will know. So the following exercises will help prepare your legs, hips, spine and mind for the sitting. Levitation comes later.

* Ideally while levitating.

What You Need:

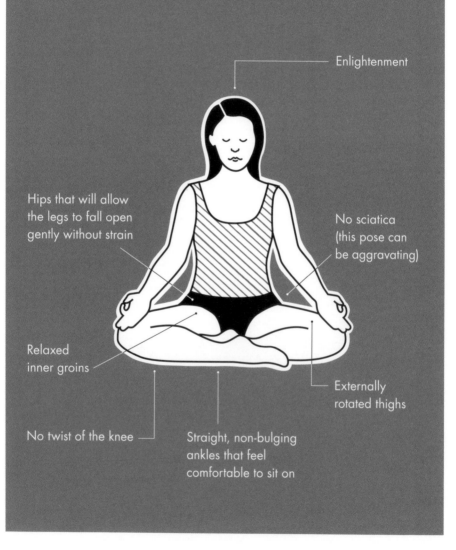

Enlightenment

Hips that will allow the legs to fall open gently without strain

No sciatica (this pose can be aggravating)

Relaxed inner groins

Externally rotated thighs

No twist of the knee

Straight, non-bulging ankles that feel comfortable to sit on

Gateway Poses

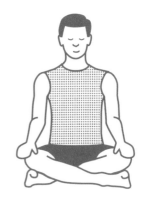

SUKHASANA
Easy pose

EQUIPMENT: A yoga brick or a yoga blanket
SUBSTITUTION OPTIONS: Folded sheets/
normal blankets/books to sit on

It's like they were named to wind you up. Sukhasana, or Easy pose, is anything but for people used to sitting on chairs. Which is basically all of us. But it is an excellent and accessible way for most people to start sitting for longer periods of time.

The majority of people will need to sit on something (not a chair) to perform this pose comfortably. This could be relatively low, like a folded blanket, or it could be a brick, a block or a cushion.

Whichever way, take something fairly comfortable to sit on, place it under your butt, and sit close to the front edge of it with your legs out straight in front of you. Use this moment to check you have chosen an appropriate height – mainly, if you feel like you're falling backwards and do not have a right angle at the hip joint, you may need to add a little more height.

Once you're satisfied with your position, bend your knees, cross your shins, and try to slip each foot under the opposite knee, making sure the ankles are comfortable. There's no need to draw the feet in towards you in this seated variation, in fact you're looking to keep them under the knees as much as possible, which is quite a way away from the pelvis. →

Check again that you can sit up straight without gripping at the hips or falling backwards. Press the sides of the feet lightly into the ground and make sure your ankles are not bending at a funky sideways angle. Let your legs be heavy and rest your hands in your lap or on your legs – palms can face up or down. Lengthen the tailbone to the floor and lift the crown of the head lightly up.

If your knees insist on staying pretty high and won't relax down, you probably have yourself a pair of pretty tight hips (any of the hip-related gateway poses in this book will help with that) or a very stressed-out body. Try to relax the hips with each breath and you may find they slowly drop the longer you sit.

Sit here for 1 minute, working up to 10 minutes, and perhaps eventually to 30 minutes. If you start to practise this pose often, make sure you alternate the crossing of the legs.

When you come out of the pose, stretch the legs out long in front of you again for a few breaths.

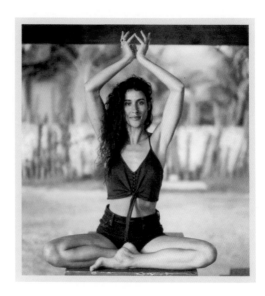

ADHO MUKHA SUKHASANA

Downward-facing Easy pose

EQUIPMENT: A yoga brick or a yoga blanket
SUBSTITUTION OPTIONS: Folded sheets/normal blankets/books to sit on

This is a nice one to work into the hips and a little into the lower back.

Start in Easy pose, sitting on whatever height works for you, and then take your fingertips to the ground in front of you, and start to fold forward (do think 'forward' rather than 'downward'). Stretch the hands away from you on the floor, ground your sit bones (try not to let the butt get light), and allow the lower back to stretch.

If your forehead reaches the floor you can rest it there. If not, take something to rest your head on – perhaps a brick or a folded blanket, so that you can relax the neck and allow the mind to be a little stiller.

Hold for 5 to 10 breaths, then slowly walk the hands back towards you, stretch the legs out long, and then change the cross of the legs and take the other side.

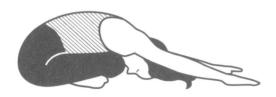

JANU SIRSASANA A

Head-to-knee pose

EQUIPMENT: A yoga brick or a yoga blanket and a strap
SUBSTITUTION OPTIONS: Folded sheets/normal blankets/books to sit on;
a belt/a tie

This is a great one for working on hip rotation (or working out how little of it you have) in order to ground the front shin bone when the leg is bent up towards you. This action is needed in both legs simultaneously in Siddhasana to keep the knees and ankles safe, so it's a good idea to practise it one leg at a time.

Start seated, possibly on height (bricks/books/blankets again – whichever option works for you), making sure that you can sit upright and your lumbar is not collapsing back behind you. Have your legs stretched out in front of you to work out what height, if any, you need.

When you've arranged yourself, keep your left leg extended in front of you, bend up your right leg and open the knee wide. Try to place your right heel as close to your upper right thigh as you can – in the groin if that's available. Make sure you externally rotate strongly from the right hip (use your butt to do this), so that you're aiming for your right shin bone – the top of it – to be placed on the floor (rather than the outer side of your calf). Think of the same action of opening the inner knee (or the knee-pit) as in Baddha Konasana (p. 155) – activating the side glutes to find space.

Your right foot traditionally points forward to the front of your mat, but if this is tricky at the ankle, it can point a little towards the left. Whichever way, make sure your ankle isn't bending sideways.

If your knee is hovering a long way off the floor: firstly, you know you need to work a little on your rotation and hip openness; secondly, place a brick under it so that your knee doesn't try to move sideways as you fold.

Inhale to lengthen your spine and on an exhale fold forward and take your left foot in your hands, or take hold of a strap looped around your left foot. Inhale to make a concave shape with your upper back, lifting the inner elbows and pulling on the foot/strap, and exhale to fold forward over your extended leg, still actively using the arms and keeping the elbows high.

Ground your sit bones and make sure your hips are in line with one another (i.e. don't let one hip draw back further than the other; usually it's the bent-leg hip that will want to sway back). Press the lumbar spine forwards but don't stick your butt out behind you; allow the lower spine to stretch up and forwards.

Breathe and hold for 5 breaths. To release, sit up, free your bent leg and straighten it out alongside your left. Rest before taking the other side.

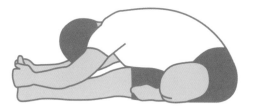

ASHWINI MUDRA

Horse gesture

This is when you get to practise
levitation, through a combination
of Pranayama (breathing exercises)
and Bandha (physical and energetic locks).
There are a few different variations of
this exercise, but this one should help you
get to grips with both the breathing and
the physical/energetic locks without
causing anxiety (but if it does,
please stop straight away).

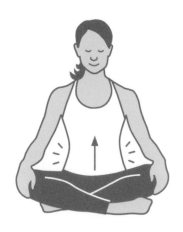

Find a seat, perhaps again in Sukhasana, with any props you need.
Allow yourself a few moments to notice your breathing, taking a few
deeper breaths in and out through the nose. When you are ready to
begin, breathe in through the nose and hold the breath at the top.
While you hold with your lungs full, engage the muscles around the anal
sphincter and pelvic floor/perineum and lift them. Draw the muscles on
and up and then release them, then engage again and then release,
imagining you're drawing energy up from the base of your spine towards
the crown of your head. Repeat this as a slow pulsing action of Mula
Bandha (the energy lock around the pelvic floor) as many times as is
comfortable, until you feel you need to release your breath. When you
need to let go, release the muscles, the Bandha, and breathe out.

Repeat this 3 to 5 times, resting as long as you need to in between.
Try to hold the breath a little longer each time if possible, but not so long
that you are gasping for breath when you breathe out. You can also play
with the speed of the pulses. In some traditions, men hold the Bandha
on for 4 seconds and women 5; in others the pulse is quicker and more
rhythmic, though never fast. See if the speed makes a difference for you,
but always keep focussing on the idea of lifting, of ascending energy.

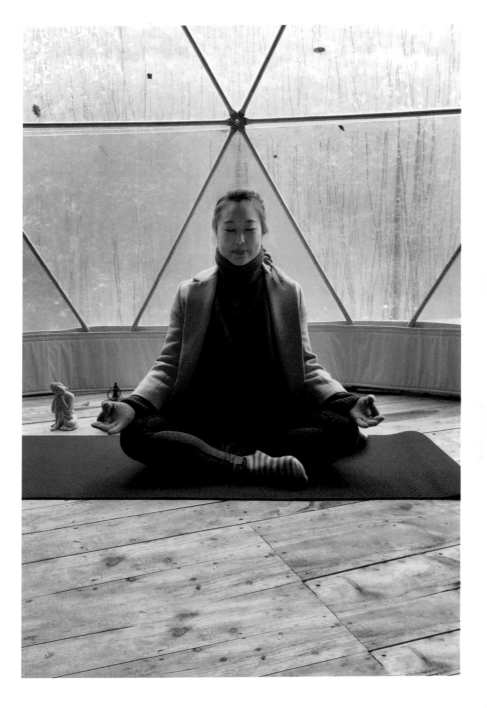

MINDFULNESS MEDITATION

As unphotogenic as it sadly is, the entire point of asana – of yoga poses – is to be able to sit, focus the mind and meditate in an ongoing way. So before you start trying to meditate in potentially less than comfortable positions with all of the physical distractions that can bring, practise your meditation in a less physically stressful way.

You can sit on a cushion with your legs crossed; you can kneel with a whole pile of cushions underneath you so that the weight of your body on your calves doesn't send them to sleep; or you can sit in a chair, ideally with a straight back and both feet on the floor. Whatever allows you to be comfortable enough, but not so comfortable that you fall asleep.

Once you have found your seat, close the eyes and start to focus on the breath. If you would rather not close the eyes you can do this with the eyes open, just try not to take in visual information – keep the focus soft and take the gaze internally.

Start by noticing the place where your breath is most physically obvious. This might be the tip of the nose or the nostrils, it could be the back of the throat or maybe the rise and fall of the chest. Wherever the breath is most present, try to hook your attention to it and observe. Notice how subtly different every single breath actually is. And notice how little time elapses before your mind wanders.

This, by the way, is exactly what everyone's mind (with the exception of the Dalai Lama) will do. Your aim is not to shut your mind up, but to observe its wandering, notice when you get caught up in thought, let it go, and return to watching your breath. You may have to do this every 5 seconds, you may have to do this every single second; the important thing is that you notice, you let go, and you get back to your focus.

Start by sitting for 10 minutes if you can, keeping up this process. You can meditate on breath, you can meditate on rising and falling sensations in the body, or you can meditate on why you feel the compulsion to perform and photograph all of the poses you've done so far.

A great starting place is 10 minutes a day. Work up to 30 over time if possible.

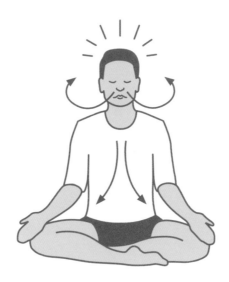

Step by Step:

HOW TO SIDDHASANA

You've opened your hips, you've released your hips, you've arranged your pelvis, you've ascended your energy and you've meditated. Now is the time to combine them all in Siddhasana.

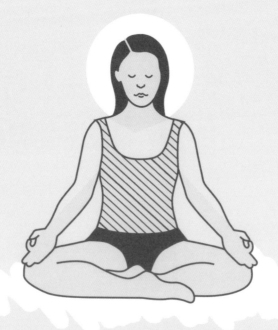

1. Start once again by sitting on a folded blanket or brick with your legs stretched out in front of you. Arrange your props so that you have roughly a right angle at the hip joint, there is no gripping of the groins, and you don't feel like you're falling backwards.

2. Bend up your left leg, opening the knee wide, and take your heel in towards your pubic bone.

3. Externally rotate strongly from the left hip, using the outer butt, and try to get the front shin on the floor (rather than the side of the calf).

4. Now draw in your right leg, opening the knee wide, externally rotating from the hip and place your right foot in front of or perhaps on top of your left foot. If it feels comfortable, you can tuck your right toes in the space between your left calf muscle and thigh.

5. Keep the spine long and upright, keep the knee-pits open and the shin bones down. Sit tall and breathe.

TAKING IT TO THE NEXT LEVEL

Other than increasing your daily meditation to 12 hours, you can of course learn to levitate and reach samadhi: yogic bliss.

#Instatips

With all the posing that abounds, it's important to make sure that other people know you have a non-ego side, and that much of your practice – despite all apparent Insta evidence to the contrary – is in fact silent reflection and meditation. So make sure your grid contains at least one picture of your very personal and private daily, silent meditative retreat pose.

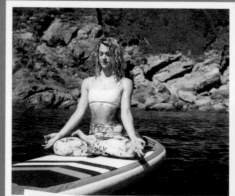

LOCATION, LOCATION, LOCATION

A pose like Siddhasana is well suited to nature. Perhaps sit on a tree stump surrounded by leaves, trunks and shrubs, or in a countrified, specially built yoga shala, surrounded by asymmetric beams and dome structures.

The ultimate location, of course, is somewhere that literally allows you to float. Consider being on water for your levitating meditation pose.

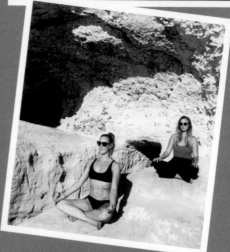

COSTUME

Make sure you go 'make-up-free'. And by this I mean wearing as much make-up as you need to give yourself the dewy, rosy-cheeked look of not wearing any make-up. If you still look like you're wearing make-up, take it off, but apply a serious filter to your pic to make your face look manageable. Ensure you let everyone know how #brave you are for going #makeupless by adding all the #raw #real #unfiltered hashtags.

PROPS

All of nature is your prop. Meditating outside is handy not only for the natural surroundings, but it also shows your commitment, especially if it is cold.

Also, consider surrounding yourself with the material trappings of spiritualism – Buddha statues, beads, Indian deities, tiny cymbals – all those things you never knew existed until you stepped into your favourite yoga studio.

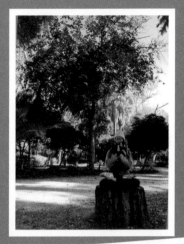

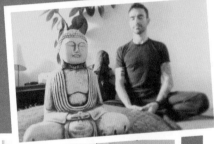

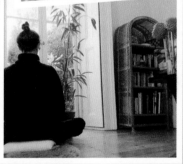

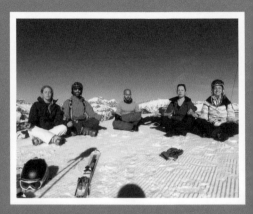

DANGER RATING

The danger in this photo is in disturbing your perfectly manicured Insta garden with a picture of your actual self. If you want to keep your Insta-influencer crown, this can be a tricky one to pull off. Due to danger of being unfollowed (which is in itself a little death), this has a rating of 9.

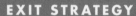

EXIT STRATEGY

Apply make-up. Breathe a sigh of relief. Get on with your handstands/day.

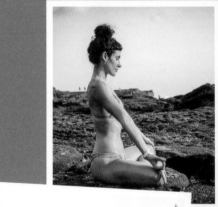

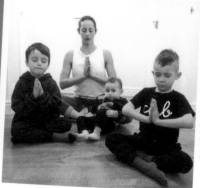

#NSFL

(NOT SAFE FOR LIFE)

It is, of course, possible to combine the no-clothes rule,
the meditating-in-the-great-outdoors-in-the-cold commitment
with the beard AND the tattoos. Then you get this. Insta-win.

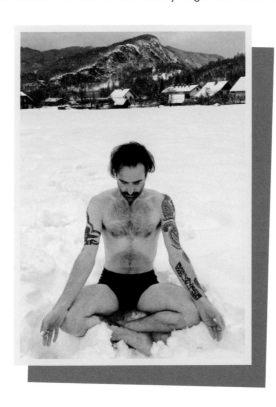

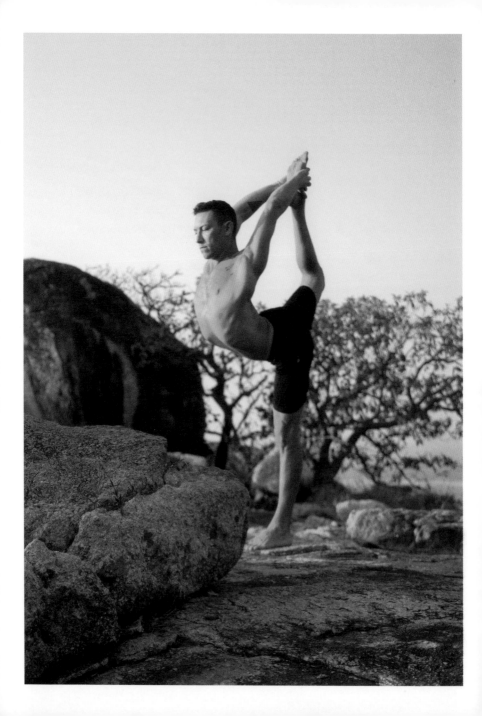

Epilogue: Closing thoughts

Coming out of your final meditation pose, you might, for a moment, feel a little reflective over the time you've spent grunting, sweating, and negotiating the angle of the sun at 3pm on a Tuesday on a Goan beach to find your perfect shot.

Perhaps you found a new focus through working on the postures. Perhaps you found a sweet moment of stillness in the briefest of balances. Perhaps you even learnt something about your tenacity in the face of a challenge or, gradually, your ability to let things go (unless they're Insta followers. Never let go of Insta followers).

Of course, every pose that you work so hard to achieve will eventually leave you, no matter how long it took you to practise it or photograph it. Some people even suggest there may come a time when Instagram is no longer the ultimate hub of human existence. Though this seems unlikely.

Part of your practice therefore, is learning to let go – of yoga postures, frustrations, ambitions, timescales, ideas, comparisons and, ultimately, your selfie. Postures will come and go, pictures will win and fail, and sometimes the Insta lives of others you covet might not prove entirely reflective of their truth. Learning to accept these things, to change what you can and let go of what you can't is what the practice is all about. Yoga is about that realisation that you are enough just as you are; it just helps if you're in a bikini #yogaforthewin.

GLOSSARY

PROTRACTION: the action of extending a part of the body often by drawing things apart (for instance, in the case of the shoulder blades, drawing them away from one another)

RETRACTION: the action of drawing something back in (for instance, drawing the shoulder blades together)

JOINT HYPER-EXTENSION: to move a joint beyond its 'normal' range of motion (e.g. elbows that bend backwards or knees that swing backwards)

FLEXION: the action of bending, usually towards the midline (e.g. bringing the knee to the chest is flexion of the hip joint)

EXTENSION: the action of straightening a limb or stretching away from the midline (e.g. stretching your leg out behind you is extension at the hip joint)

EXTERNAL ROTATION: to rotate outwards (away from the midline)

INTERNAL ROTATION: to rotate inwards (towards the midline)

ELEVATION: to raise up

DEPRESSION: to drop down

CLOSING THE RIBS: drawing the lower ribs lightly towards each other

LORDOSIS: a pronounced inward curve of the lower (lumbar) spine

KYPHOSIS: a pronounced outward curve in the upper (thoracic) spine

ASANA: yoga postures

MARCUS VEDA
is a yoga teacher and DJ.
He is renowned for breaking
down difficult poses and
pushing people to their edge
– with a good dose of fun.

HANNAH WHITTINGHAM
is a yoga teacher, writer
and magician's assistant who
can be found strengthening
limbs of yogis across London,
or bending her own into
magic boxes.

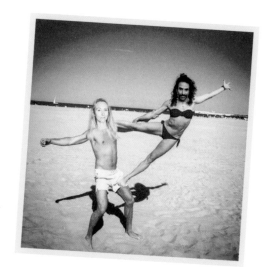

PHOTOGRAPHIC ACKNOWLEDGEMENTS

A genuine and unsarcastic big bucket of thank-yous to our friends and
fellow yogis of London and beyond, who allowed us to use their pictures
in the full knowledge that we would be mercilessly lampooning the
entire world of Instayoga. The very fact that you agreed is testament to
your openness, humour and generosity. We are deeply flattered and
appreciative of your trust in us and, especially, in a book about which we
could give you so little detail. Thank you. We love you. You are awesome.

David Pearce / Lita Sattva / Emily Mergaert / Alan Ellman / Katarina
Rayburn / Natasha Cornish / Nicki Ratcliffe / Dav Jones / Wen-Chuan Dai
/ Cheryl Teagann / Jonelle Lewis / Raj Chande / Sylvia Garcia / Adam
King / Kimbal Quist Bumstead / Tom Berry / Maxim Lucas / Phoenix Veda
/ Ana Dias / Samuel Nwokeka / Rory Moody / Helen Russell Clark /
Rachel Mills / Joe Adams / Juan Montoliu / Leon London / Tom Holmes
/ Isabel Lankester / Natasha Veda / Steven Zwerink / Ambra Vallo

10 9 8 7 6 5 4 3 2 1

Vermilion, an imprint of Ebury Publishing,
20 Vauxhall Bridge Road,
London, SW1V 2SA

Vermilion is part of the Penguin Random House group of companies whose
addresses can be found at global.penguinrandomhouse.com

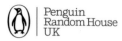
Penguin
Random House
UK

Text copyright © Hannah Whittingham and Marcus Veda
Photography © see photo credits on page 191

Hannah Whittingham and Marcus Veda have asserted their right to be
identified as the authors of this Work in accordance with the Copyright,
Designs and Patents Act 1988

First published by Vermilion in 2019

www.penguin.co.uk

A CIP catalogue record for this book is available from the British Library

Design: Louise Evans
Photography: see photo credits on page 191

ISBN: 9781785042478
Colour Reproduction by Altaimage London Ltd
Printed and bound in China by C&C Offset Printing Co., Ltd.

Penguin Random House is committed to a sustainable future for
our business, our readers and our planet. This book is made from
Forest Stewardship Council® certified paper.

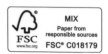

Hannah and Marcus are also the authors of *Greed, Sex, Intention:
Living Like a Yogi in the 21st Century*, in which they attempt to drag
3,000-year-old ethics into the modern world.